ॐ

MARMA POINTS OF SUSHRUTA

the foundation of Modern Kinesiology

Ashwini Kumar Aggarwal

जय गुरुदेव

ISBN13: 978-93-95766-06-7 Paperback Edition
ISBN13: 978-93-95766-07-4 Hardbound Edition
ISBN13: 978-93-95766-08-1 Digital Edition

Title: **Marma Points of Sushruta the foundation of Modern Kinesiology**
Author: **Ashwini Kumar Aggarwal**

Printed and Published by
Devotees of Sri Sri Ravi Shankar Ashram
34 Sunny Enclave, Devigarh Road
Patiala 147001, Punjab, India

https://advaita56.weebly.com/
The Art of Living Centre

https://www.artofliving.org/

26th Sep 2022 Monday, Shukla Paksha Pratipada, Sharad Ritu, Navratri begins, Ashwin Masa, Hasta Nakshatra, Dakshinayana, Ghatasthapana (Kalash Sthapan), Maharaja Agrasen Jayanti
On this day in 1946 Tintin by Herge is published, 1957 Dag Hammarskjold reelected Secretary-General of UN, 1973 Concorde Jet makes first transatlantic crossing, 1980 Soyuz 38 spaceflight returns from Salyut 6 spacestation.
Vikram Samvat 2079 Nala, Saka Era 1944 Shubhakrit

1st Edition September 2022

जय गुरुदेव

Dedication

Sri Sri Ravi Shankar

who rediscovers our ancient practices and makes them global effortlessly

Blessing

All the sensory nerves end in the tip of the nose. There are two points that are important for alertness and focus of the brain - the ear lobes and tip of the nose. They are the **marma** points. These are the secret points. If you keep your attention on the tip of the nose, your focus improves, especially for children.

Sri Sri Ravi Shankar
Advance Course Talks

Acknowledgements

17th Sep 2022 Lord's fabulous satsang at Guru Paduka vanam honoring Assam CM and India's PM, with Anuj Urvee + their papa mummy. A grateful Calcutta couple hands their checklist to Gurudev. On 18th a 40min meditation at Gurupadukavanam by Gurudev based on Yama Niyama of Patanjali. Gurudev's delicate touch on 19th evening at Ganga Kutir. 25th Sep mummy Mahalaya Amavasya pitr annadan + gau puja.

Cover Photo Credits

Photo by Marcos Gael Martínez from Pexels:
https://www.pexels.com/photo/black-and-white-photo-of-a-graceful-woman-ballet-dancer-17029022/

Preface

```
During a trek to virgin nature in the midst of an Advanced Meditation Program,
  • the body becomes incredibly fit.
  • Unbelievable insights open up in the mind.
  • The family stops complaining.
  • The heart gets filled with love.
And the Lord smiles and showers bliss.
```

Marma is the father of Prana management. There are many techniques in use today that help direct the flow of consciousness in the body, that in turn release blocks and cause massive healing to occur.

Some of the common forks of Marma include:

- Acupressure and acupuncture
- Polarity routines
- Reiki
- Reflexology
- Meru Chikitsa
- Osteopathy
- Meditation in Motion
- CranioSacral Therapy (CST)
- Massage
- Touch

Prana is the vital life force. It is that energy within the body that is directly linked to the soul. The supreme consciousness or Brahman manifests in each being and body as a glow of light. This light is not exactly "photon". It is something subtle, that cannot be grasped by the senses, nor by the intellect, but it can be felt strongly in emotions like cheerfulness, strength, vitality, enthusiasm, love, joy, stamina, forgiveness, compassion.

Marma therapy works on this **light body**. Marma point are simply those points within the body where the chances of this light being hindered or disturbed are quite high. When the light or glow within a being gets upset or scattered, it manifests as a weakness that is sensed as guilt, fear, illness, pain, bitterness, grief or brokenness. Simple by gentle touch, meditation, massage, carefree laughter, a long walk or a proper bath, the **light being** gets restored and immense healing happens.

The current scope of this book is limited to the method of gentle touch at the Marma points, as outlined in the ancient Ayurvedic text named Sushruta Samhita.

Table of Contents

BLESSING 4

PREFACE 5

PRAYER 10

ETYMOLOGY OF WORD MARMA 11

THE 7 DHATUS OF ANATOMICAL BODY 12

THE 7 LAYERS OF EXISTENCE 12

THE 7 CHAKRAS AND MARMA POINTS 13

THE 3 PRINCIPAL NADIS 15

ANGULA MEASUREMENTS 15

SUSHRUTA SAMHITA - MARMA VERSES 16

Body Location wrt Marma Point Name 17
Leg and Foot Marma Point Names (paired) 18
Chest and Abdomen Marma Point Names 22
Back Marma Point Names (paired) 24
Arm and Hand Marma Point Names (paired) 26
Head and Neck Marma Point Names 30
Body Tissue type wrt Marma Point Name 45
Body Injurious Condition wrt Marma Point Name 47
Definition of Marma 50

SUSHRUTA'S 107 MARMA POINTS ANATOMICALLY GROUPED 44+12+14+37 51

Dhamani Matrika Shringataka Simanta Marma Points 56
Dimensions of each of Sushruta's 107 Marma Points 57

SUSHRUTA'S 107 MARMA POINTS COLLATED 60

ASHTANGA HRIDAYAM OF VAGBHATTA - MARMA VERSES 69

CHARAKA SAMHITA - MARMA VERSES 72

107 MARMA POINTS ALPHABETICAL WRT BODY ANATOMY 73

107 MARMA POINTS ANATOMICAL DISTRIBUTION HEAD TO TOE 75

Discrete Points in Midline Vertical Axis of body = (1x6)+1 = 7 76
107. Adhipati (Brahmarandhra) Features 77
97. Sthapani Features 77
77. Matrika2a (Kanthanadi) Features 78
48. Hridaya Features 78
47. Nabhi Features 79
46. Basti Features 79
45. Guda Features 80
Discrete Points in Skull = 1x5 = 5 81
106. Simanta5 (Manyamula) Features 84
105. Simanta4 (Shivarandhra) Features 84
104. Simanta3 (Vishnurandhra) Features 85
103. Simanta2 (Kapala) Features 85
102. Simanta1 (Nasamula) Features 86

PAIR POINTS IN FACE = 4+(5X2) = 14 ... 87
101. Shringataka 4a,b (Kaninaka) Features ... 89
100. Shringataka 3a,b (Karnapali) Features ... 89
99. Shringataka 2a,b (Kapolanasa) Features ... 90
98. Shringataka 1a,b (Oshtha, Hanu) Features ... 90
95,96. Utkshepa Features ... 91
93,94. Shankha Features ... 91
91,92. Avarta Features ... 92
89,90. Apanga Features ... 92
87,88. Phana Features ... 93
PAIR POINTS IN NECK = 8X2 -1 = 15 ... 94
85,86. Vidhura Features ... 95
83,84. Krikatika Features ... 95
81,82. Matrika 4a,4b (manyāmaṇi, grīvā) Features ... 96
79,80. Matrika 3a,3b (pṛṣṭhagrīva) Features ... 96
78. Matrika 2b (kaṇṭha) Features ... 97
75,76. Matrika 1a,1b (Akshaka) Features ... 97
73,74. Dhamani Manya Features ... 98
71,72. Dhamani Nila Features ... 98
PAIR POINTS IN BACK = 7X2 = 14 ... 99
69,70. Amsa Features ... 100
67,68. Amsaphalaka Features ... 100
65,66. Brihati Features ... 101
63,64. Parshvasandhi Features ... 101
61,62. Nitamba Features ... 102
59,60. Kukundara Features ... 102
57,58. Katikataruna Features ... 103
PAIR POINTS IN CHEST = 4X2 = 8 ... 104
55,56. Apastambha Features ... 105
53,54. Apalapa Features ... 105
51,52. Stanarohita Features ... 106
49,50. Stanamula Features ... 106
PAIR POINTS IN ARMS = 7X2 = 14 ... 107
43,44. Kakshadhara Features ... 108
41,42. Lohitaksha Arm Features ... 108
39,40. Urvi Arm Features ... 109
37,38. Ani Arm Features ... 109
35,36. Kurpara Features ... 110
33,34. Indrabasti Arm Features ... 110
31,32. Manibandha Features ... 111
PAIR POINTS IN HANDS = 4X2 = 8 ... 112
29,30. Kurchashira Hand Features ... 113
27,28. Kurcha Hand Features ... 113
25,26. Talahridaya Hand Features ... 114
23,24. Kshipra Hand Features ... 114
PAIR POINTS AT GENITALS = 2X2 = 4 ... 115
21,22. Vitapa Features ... 116
19,20. Lohitaksha Leg Features ... 116
PAIR POINTS IN LEGS = 5X2 = 10 ... 117
17,18. Urvi Leg Features ... 118
15,16. Ani Leg Features ... 118
13,14. Janu Features ... 119

11,12. Indrabasti Leg Features ... 119
9,10. Gulpha Features ... 120
Pair Points in Feet = 4x2 = 8 ... 121
7,8. Kurchashira Feet Features ... 122
5,6. Kurcha Feet Features ... 122
3,4. Talahridaya Feet Features ... 123
1,2. Kshipra Feet Features ... 123

GLOWING BODY AND CONSCIOUSNESS ... 124

BIOLUMINESCENT BODY AND MARMA ... 125

SIMPLY EFFECTIVE MARMA THERAPY TECHNIQUES ... 126

Barefoot Walking ... 126
Oiled Clapping ... 126
Boisterous Laughter ... 126
Eating together ... 126
Guided Meditation ... 126
Yoganidra ... 126
Showering Properly ... 126
Dipping feet in lukewarm water with Rocksalt ... 126
Palming the Eyes ... 127
Shirodhara and Abhyanga Panchakarma ... 127
Mountain Trekking ... 127
Listening to a Rudram Chant ... 127
Applying Henna Mehandi ... 127

A TRADITIONAL MARMA CHIKITSA PROTOCOL ... 128

POLARITY ROUTINE ... 129
Changeover using YOUTH MUDRA ... 131
TOUCH ROUTINE ... 132

WHICH? SUGGESTED OILS MEDITATION ... 134

NOTES FROM PERSONAL MARMA SESSIONS ... 135

ETYMOLOGY OF WORD AYURVEDA ... 137

LATIN TRANSLITERATION CHART ... 138

MARMA POINTS LIST ... 139

INDEX OF MARMA POINTS SANSKRIT ... 141

INDEX OF MARMA POINTS ENGLISH ... 143

FEW MARMA POINTS NAMED VARIOUSLY ... 145

REFERENCES ... 146

EPILOGUE ... 148

Table of Figures

Figure 1 Marma Points in vertical midline axis of Body 13
Figure 2: Marma Points wrt 7 Chakras (Patanjali) 14
Figure 3 Marma Points in Feet 18
Figure 4 Marma Points in Legs and Feet 19
Figure 5 Marma Points in Leg and Foot (Side View) 20
Figure 6 Marma Points in Legs and Feet (Posterior View) 21
Figure 7 Marma Point Guda 22
Figure 8 Marma Points in Chest and Abdomen 23
Figure 9 Marma Points in Back 25
Figure 10 Marma Points in Hands 26
Figure 11 Marma Points in Arms and Hands 27
Figure 12 Marma Points in Hands 28
Figure 13 Marma Points in Arms wrt Feet 29
Figure 14 Marma Points in Throat (Neck Front View) 31
Figure 15 Marma Points in Neck (Rear View) 32
Figure 16 Marma Points in Neck (Side View) 33
Figure 17 Marma Points in Face except shringataka 34
Figure 18 Marma Points in Face (Side View) except shringataka 35
Figure 19 Marma Points Shringataka on 4 Sense Organ Nerves 36
Figure 20 Marma Points Shringataka on 4 Sense Organ Nerves in Practice 37
Figure 21 Marma Points on Face in Practice 38
Figure 22 Marma Points on Skull (Top View) 39
Figure 23 Marma Practice Points on Skull (Top View) 40
Figure 24 Marma Points Simanta five nos and Adhipati (Left Side View) 41
Figure 25 Marma Points Simanta and Adhipati (Right Side View) 42
Figure 26 Marma Points on Skull in Practice 43
Figure 27 Marma Points Simanta (Front View) 44
Figure 28 Marma Points Simanta (Rear View) 44
Figure 29 Marma Points Whole Body (Front View – Points of Back are not here) 61
Figure 30 Marma Points Whole Body (Rear View) 63
Figure 31 Marma Points Whole Body Front View (Upper Half) 65
Figure 32 Marma Points Whole Body Front View (Lower Half) 66
Figure 33 Marma Points Whole Body Rear View (Upper Half) 67
Figure 34 Marma Points Whole Body Rear View (Lower Half) 68
Figure 35: Marma Points Midline Vertical Axis 76
Figure 36: Schematic of Skull (Top View) 81
Figure 37: Marma Points in Skull (Top View) 82
Figure 38: Marma Points in Skull (Back View) 83
Figure 39: Marma Points in Face (Front View) 87
Figure 40: Marma Points in Face (Side View) 88
Figure 41: Marma Points in Neck (Front View) 94
Figure 42: Marma Points in Back 99
Figure 43: Marma Points in Chest except those already accounted for 104

Prayer

ॐ

नमामि धन्वन्तरिम् आदि देवम् ।
सुरासुरैर् वन्दित पाद-पद्मम् ॥

लोके जरा-रुक्- भय-मृत्यु-नाशम् ।
धातारमीशम् विविधौषधीनाम् ॥

oṃ

namāmi dhanvantarim ādi devam I

surāsurair vandita pāda-padmam II

loke jarā-ruk-bhaya-mṛtyu-nāśam I

dhātāramīśam vividhauṣadhīnām II

Om
Sincere salutations to Dhanvantari, the first among healing deities.
O Ye! Whom both the fortunate and the unfortunate extol, Ye whose lotus feet are a source of curing energies.

In this ephemeral world who

- delivers freedom from old age by rebirth
- provides solutions for diseases and lifestyle management
- banishes fear
- prevents accidental death or violent end

The divine well-wisher of all; by his various formulations, techniques, and herbs.

Etymology of word MARMA

Marma = मर्म = that which is soft, delicate, subtle, secret.

Dhatupatha Root 1403 मृ (मृङ्) प्राणत्यागे । That where the Prana moves, or escapes from. 6th conjugation.

Sanskrit Stem or Pratipadika of Marma is मर्मन् neuter.

Noun declension 7x3 Matrix.

मर्मन् n	singular	dual	plural
Vocative	मर्मन्	मर्मणी	मर्माणि
1st case	मर्म	मर्मणी	मर्माणि
2nd case	मर्म	मर्मणी	मर्माणि
3rd case	मर्मणा	मर्मभ्याम्	मर्मभिः
4th case	मर्मणे	मर्मभ्याम्	मर्मभ्यः
5th case	मर्मणः	मर्मभ्याम्	मर्मभ्यः
6th case	मर्मणः	मर्मणोः	मर्मणाम्
7th case	मर्मणि	मर्मणोः	मर्मसु

The 7 Dhatus of Anatomical Body

The science of Ayurveda or wholistic healing has grouped the anatomical body into the seven DHATUS or TISSUES, viz. रस RASA (plasma and lymph fluids) रक्त RAKTA (red blood cells), मांस MĀṂSA (muscle), मेदस् MEDAS (fat or adipose tissue), अस्थि ASTHI (bone), मज्जा MAJJĀ (bone marrow, nerves, tendons and ligaments), शुक्र ŚUKRA (semen, sperm, ovum). Marma is the place where the consciousness is strongly present in these tissues.

1. Rasa. Liquid viscous healing fluid that is controlled by body timer, mood and energy demand.
2. Rakta. That which transports oxygen and nutrition to all cells and nuclei.
3. Mamsa + Snayu. Strings and threads that help in movement, locomotion, lift and direction. Comprises of muscles, tendons, ligaments. Also, the nerves that help in sensory signals and transport.
4. Medas. Thick conglomerate of cells that store all kind of nutrition, and release them only if food intake is less.
5. Asthi. That which does not get eroded by time or weathering. Remains for countless years.
6. Majja. Spongy bone marrow that gives rise to new bones, helps in bone growth, or helps maintain bone movement.
7. Shukra. Vital sparkling, full of life. That which has the capacity to give birth. Create anew.

Marma is **that** presence of glowing consciousness/auspiciousness/divinity at a site, **which** can be **modulated** by touch, prayer, meditation and attention to **restore** full health, stamina and enthusiasm.

The 7 Layers of Existence

Gurudev has taught us in the Basic Happiness Course that there are seven layers of existence, viz. BODY BREATH MIND INTELLECT MEMORY EGO SOUL. The powerful breathing technique named **Sudarshan Kriya** of the Art of Living works on all these layers, and thus activates the Marma points and provides a wonderful blissful experience that is much sought for by all of mankind.

1. Body. That which is opaque and solid, yet contains enough space. A reflection of the cosmos.
2. Breath. That which connects, communicates with, & empowers all discrete parts of the Body.
3. Mind. That which interfaces and transacts this Body with anything outside, apart.
4. Intellect. Reason and decision making faculty, interfaces with Memory.
5. Memory. Collection of RAM ROM EEPROM HDD SSD CloudStorage. Critical for functioning.
6. Ego. That which separates this Body from the rest of Creation. Limiting line or tendency.
7. Soul. Vital sparkling, life giving. An undeciphered entity that *needs to be freed* from the clutches of Body and Mind. That which is stated as God in the Scriptures. That which is supposed to exist in every discrete entity of creation, and beyond.

The 7 Chakras and Marma Points

SNo	Chakra Name	Marma Point Name		Anatomy	Remarks
7th chakra	Sahasrāra	Adhipati	1	crown	Brahmarandhra/Mūrdhni मूर्ध्नि
6th chakra	Ājñā	Sthapani	1	3rd eye	In between the eyebrows
5th chakra	Viśuddhi	Kanthanādi	1	throat groove	1 point of 8 points - matrika 4 pairs
4th chakra	Anahata	Hridaya	1	heart area	Center of chest
3rd chakra	Maṇipura	Nabhi	1	navel	Place of birth, and the 2nd brain
2nd chakra	Svādhiṣṭhāna	Basti	1	bladder	A bit deeper, 2 angula below nabhi
1st chakra	Mūlādhāra	Guda	1	anus	Part that touches where we sit
7 Marma Points Corresponding to the 7 Chakras					

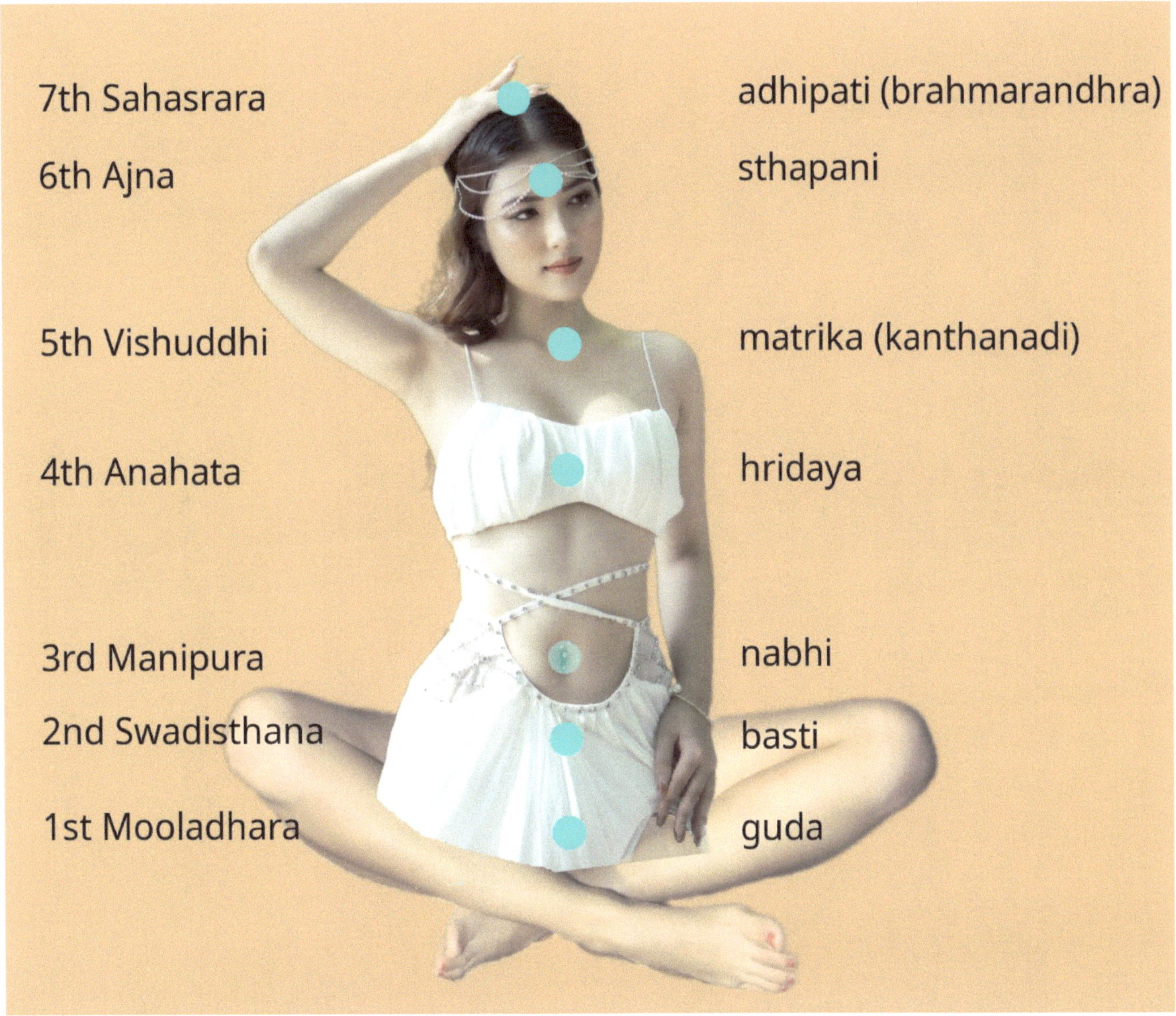

Figure 1 Marma Points in vertical midline axis of Body

Marma points of **Body Midline** corresponding to **Patanjali Yogasutras**. These reflect the **7 Major Chakras** and are the most vital points in Marma chikitsa.

SNo	Chakra Name	Marma Point Name		Patanjali	Remarks
7th chakra	Sahasrāra	Adhipati	1	मूर्धज्योतिस्	Brahmarandhra/Mūrdhni मूर्ध्नि
6th chakra	Ājñā	Sthapani	1	ज्योतिष्मती	In between the eyebrows
5th chakra	Viśuddhi	Kanthanādi	1	कण्ठकूप	1 point of 8 points - matrika 4 pairs
4th chakra	Anahata	Hridaya	1	हृदय	Center of chest
3rd chakra	Maṇipura	Nabhi	1	नाभिचक्र	Place of birth, and the 2nd brain
2nd chakra	Svādhiṣṭhāna	Basti	1	कायरूप	A bit deeper, 2 angula below nabhi
1st chakra	Mūlādhāra	Guda	1	कायाकोश	Part that touches where we sit

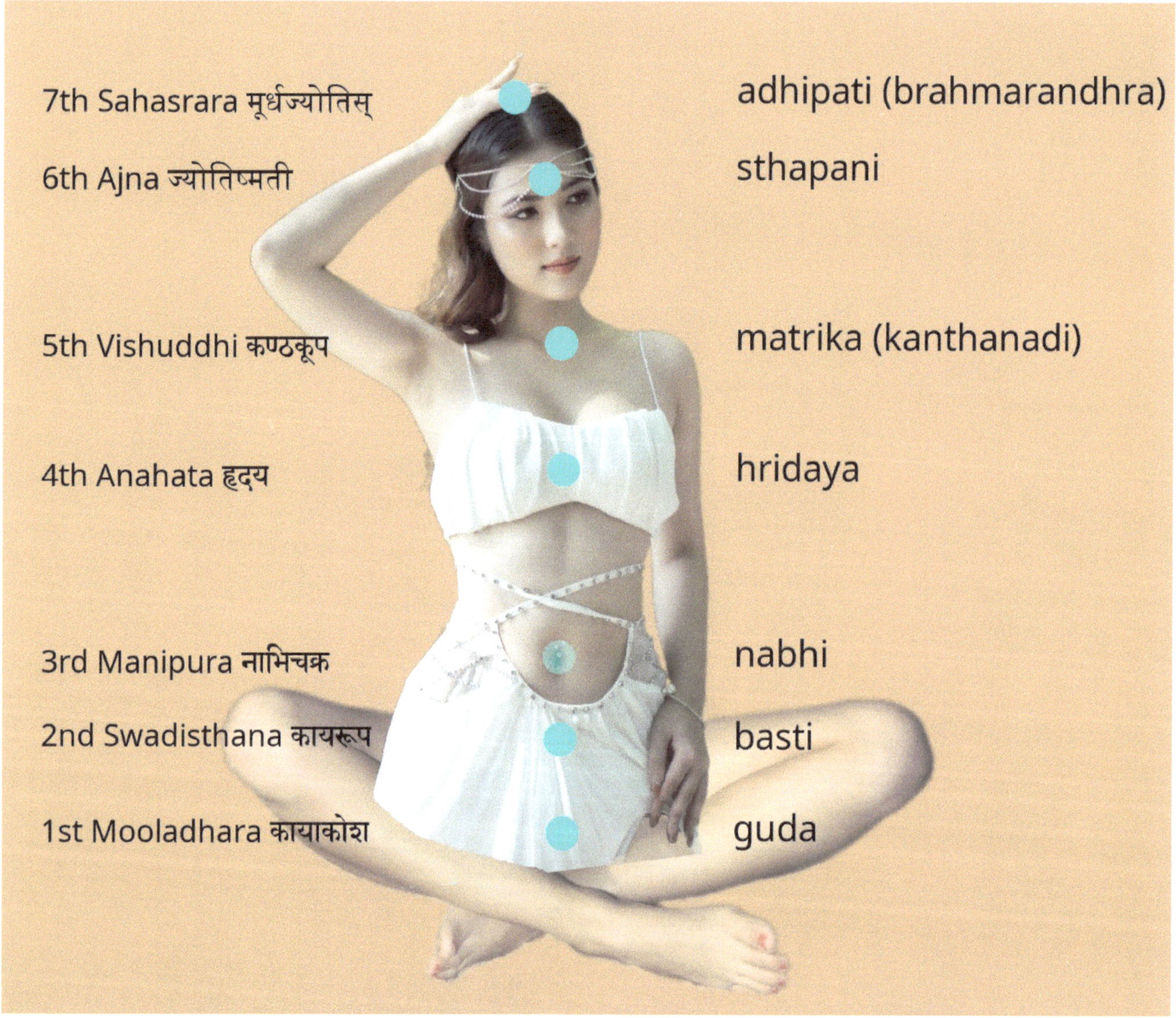

Figure 2: Marma Points wrt 7 Chakras (Patanjali)

The 3 Principal Nadis

There are the three principal nadis or subtle nerves that carry Prana flow according to the Yoga Philosophy. These are named इडा **Iḍā** (left nostril breath), पिङ्गल **Piṅgala** (right nostril breath) and सुषुम्ना **Suṣumnā** (center balanced breath).

Science has found that the breath switches every 90 seconds from the left nostril to the right, and vice versa. When the left nostril is active, processes like music, sleep, or carefree harmony get going. When the right nostril is active, processes like decision making, digestion, or selective action get success. When both nostrils are active, a sense of well-being, calmness and happiness takes over.

Yogic practices like alternate nostril breathing, switching the nostrils using specific mudras and gestures, and Meditation help enhance the success and sense of achievement. This is also the purpose of Marma Therapy.

When specific Marma points are activated, the prana flows more to these areas and organs of the body. Increased prana is responsible for healing, restoration, or repair. Increase in prana helps enhance mood and banishes fatigue, makes one more alive and receptive, and helps in wise decision-making.

e.g., When the Nabhi is massaged during a Marma session, the functioning of all organs of the abdomen, viz. stomach, duodenum, liver, spleen, gall-bladder, pancreas, kidneys and intestines; gets a major boost. These eight organs listed get superbly invigorated in eight marma sessions spread over a few months.

Angula Measurements

Angula measurement is derived from अङ्गुलि Aṅguli = Finger.

1 Angula is precisely the horizontal width of the middle segment of middle finger of a particular person. This measurement is **relative** to the body of the person, i.e., 1 angula will vary in exact size from person to person, since width of each person's finger will vary slightly.

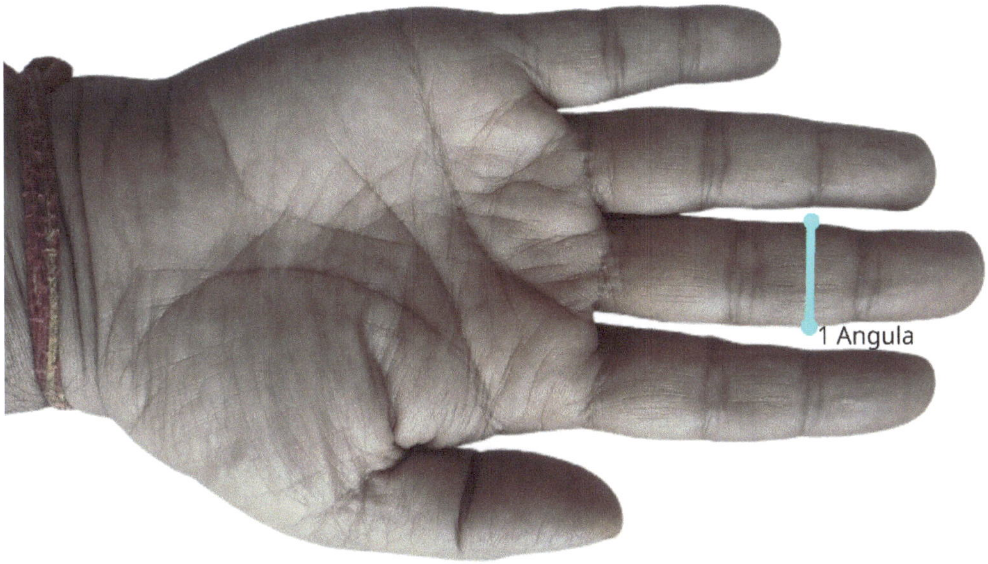

Sushruta Samhita - Marma Verses

The classic Indian text of Medicine and Surgery by the famed Rishi Sushruta consists of 40 chapters. Its 4th section is named शारीरस्थानम् Sharira Sthanam, which is a discussion and description of Human Anatomy. In this Sharira Sthanam of Sushruta Samhita, the 6th chapter is on Marma.

षष्ठोऽध्यायः ṣaṣṭho'dhyāyaḥ

६. प्रत्येकमर्मनिर्देशशारीरम् ॥ 6. pratyekamarmanirdeśaśārīram ॥

प्रत्येक-मर्म-निर्देश-शारीरोप-क्रमः ॥ Definition and precise position of each Marma point within the Human body in sequence.

अथातः प्रत्येक-मर्म-निर्देशं शारीरं व्याख्यास्यामः And now we list each of the subtle points in the body in detail ॥ १ ॥ यथोवाच भगवान् धन्वन्तरिः ॥ २ ॥ As enunciated by Lord Dhanvantri himself.
सप्तोत्तरं मर्मशतम् 107 Marma Points । तानि मर्माणि पञ्चात्मकानि भवन्ति Classified as 5 Types based on Body Tissue । तद्यथा मांसमर्माणि Mamsa Marmas, सिरामर्माणि Sira Marmas, स्नायुमर्माणि Snayu Marmas, अस्थिमर्माणि Asthi Marmas, सन्धिमर्माणि Sandhi Marmas चेति ॥ ३ ॥
न खलु मांससिरास्नाय्वस्थिसन्धिव्यतिरेकेणान्यानि मर्माणि भवन्ति । यस्मान्नोपलभ्यन्ते ॥ ४ ॥
तत्रैकादश मांसमर्माणि 11 Mamsa Marma Points, एकचत्वारिंशत् सिरामर्माणि 41 Sira Marma Points, सप्तविंशतिः स्नायुमर्माणि 27 Snayu Marma Points, अष्टावस्थिमर्माणि 8 Asthi Marma Points, विंशतिः सन्धिमर्माणि 20 Sandhi Marma Points चेति । तदेतत् सप्तोत्तरं मर्मशतम् Thus 107 total ॥ ५ ॥

Marma Body Tissues are classified as: (*Definitions solely in the context of Marma Chikitsa*)

- māṃsa = Muscles etc., such movement causing or supporting tissues
- sirā = Veins Arteries etc., such tubes, ducts, vessels or pathways
- snāyu = Nerves Ligaments Tendons etc., such attaching wires, cords, and sensation causing
- asthi = Bones Teeth Nails Hair etc., such tissues
- sandhi = Joints = where two or more bones join together

Body Location wrt Marma Point Name

तेषामेकादशैकस्मिन् सक्थ्नि भवन्ति of these 11 are in the region of one thigh and lower body parts, एतेनेतरसक्थि बाहू च व्याख्यातौ similarly 11 in one arm and hand, उदरोरसोर्द्वादश 12 are located in chest and abdomen, चतुर्दश पृष्ठे 14 are located behind, ग्रीवां प्रत्यूर्ध्वं सप्तत्रिंशत् ॥ ६ ॥ 37 are located in neck and above it.

Marma Points counted by location within the Body:

- Located in one Thigh and Lower than that = 11 (thus 11x2 = 22 Marmas in legs and feet)
- Located in one Arm and Hand = 11 (thus 11x2 = 22 Marmas in arms and hands)
- Located in Chest and Abdomen = 12
- Located behind i.e., in the Back = 14
- Located above the Clavicle i.e., in the Neck, Face, Head = 37

Leg and Foot Marma Point Names (paired)

तत्र सक्थिमर्माणि क्षिप्रतलहृदयकूर्चकूर्चशिरोगुल्फेन्द्रबस्तिजान्वाण्यूर्वीलोहिताक्षाणि विटपं चेति । (alternate reading ण्युर्वी). Thigh and lower anatomy marma points list.

तत्र सक्थि-मर्माणि क्षिप्र[1]-तलहृदय[2]-कूर्च[3]-कूर्चशिरः[4]-गुल्फ[5]-इन्द्रबस्ति[6]-जानु[7]-आणि[8]-ऊर्वी[9]-लोहिताक्षाणि[10] विटपं[11] चेति ।

- 11 viṭapa *(topmost point in this list)* = base of shoot, nerve, muscle
- 10 lohitākṣa = thigh joint, where the leg joins the torso
- 9 ūrvī (*also spelt* urvī) = middle of the thigh
- 8 āṇi = that which is at the circumference of axle
- 7 jānu = knee
- 6 indrabasti = exact center of calf, sensory bladder of lower leg that circulates blood
- 5 gulpha = ankle bone
- 4 kūrcaśira = very top of the big toe where it joins the leg
- 3 kūrca = bunch of nerves, root of big toe
- 2 talahṛdaya = heart-center of sole
- 1 kṣipra *(bottommost point in this list)* = where big toe and next toe finger meet

Literal meaning to help in comprehension/location
These points are listed in sequence of vertical location top to bottom of anatomy.

एतेनेतरत्सक्थि व्याख्यातम् । These are **mirrored** points in each leg, so a count of 22 points.

Note: Marma points **Viṭapa, Jānu** and **Gulpha** in **leg** correspond to **Kakṣadhara, Kūrpara** and **Maṇibandha** in **arm** resp.

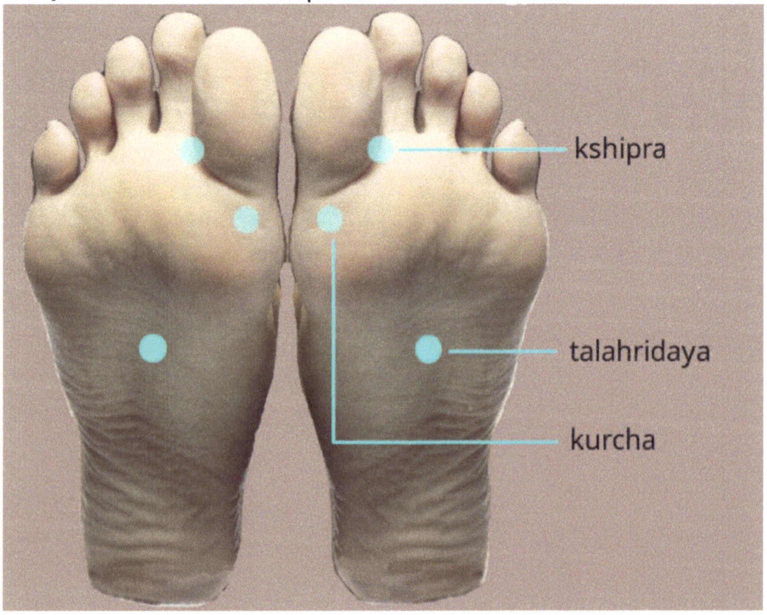

Figure 3 Marma Points in Feet

Note: Talahridaya Marma points are specifically in the sole, whereas the others are reflected both in sole and dorsum (top of foot).

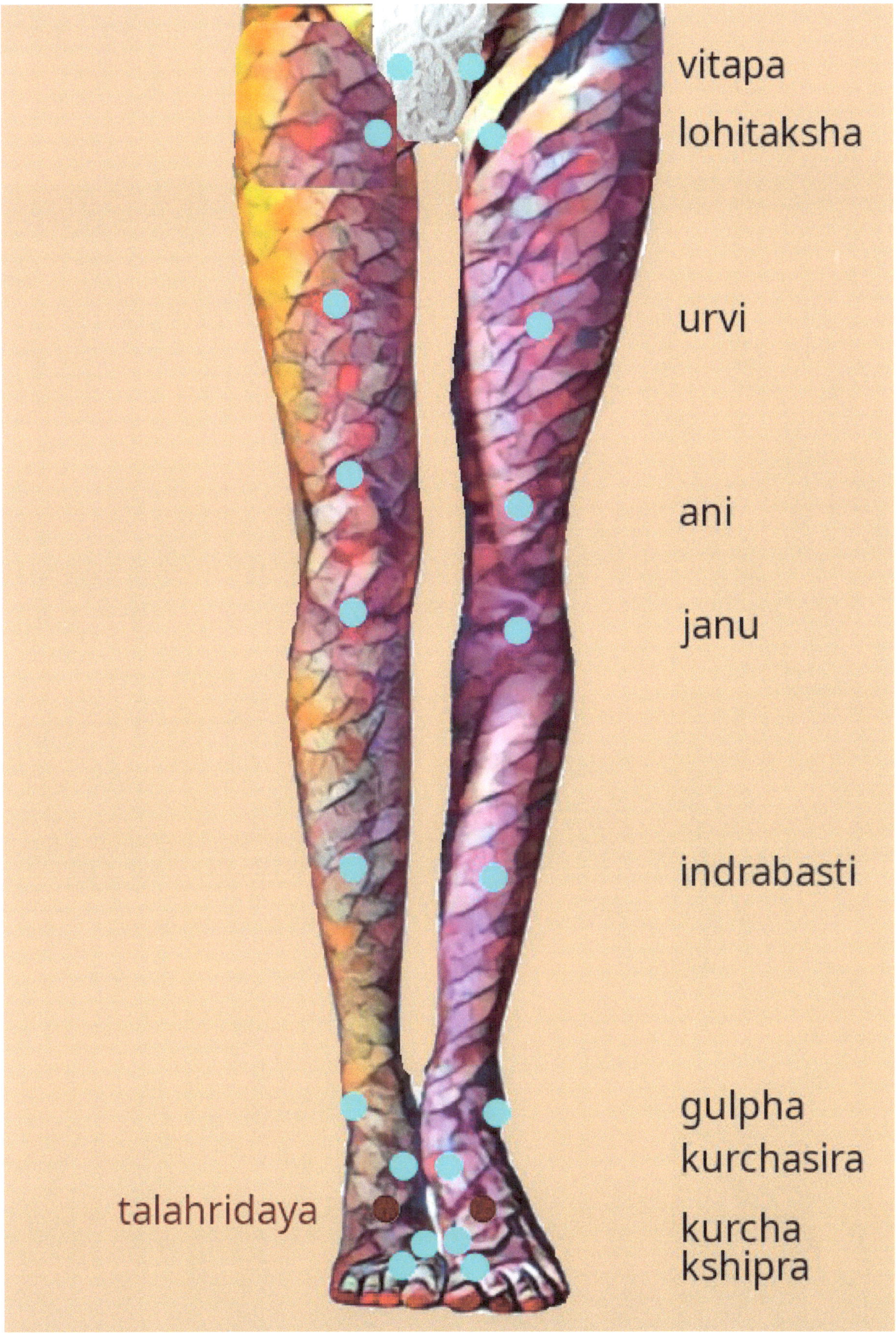

Figure 4 Marma Points in Legs and Feet

Note: Talahridaya Marma points are specifically in the sole and not the top of the foot.

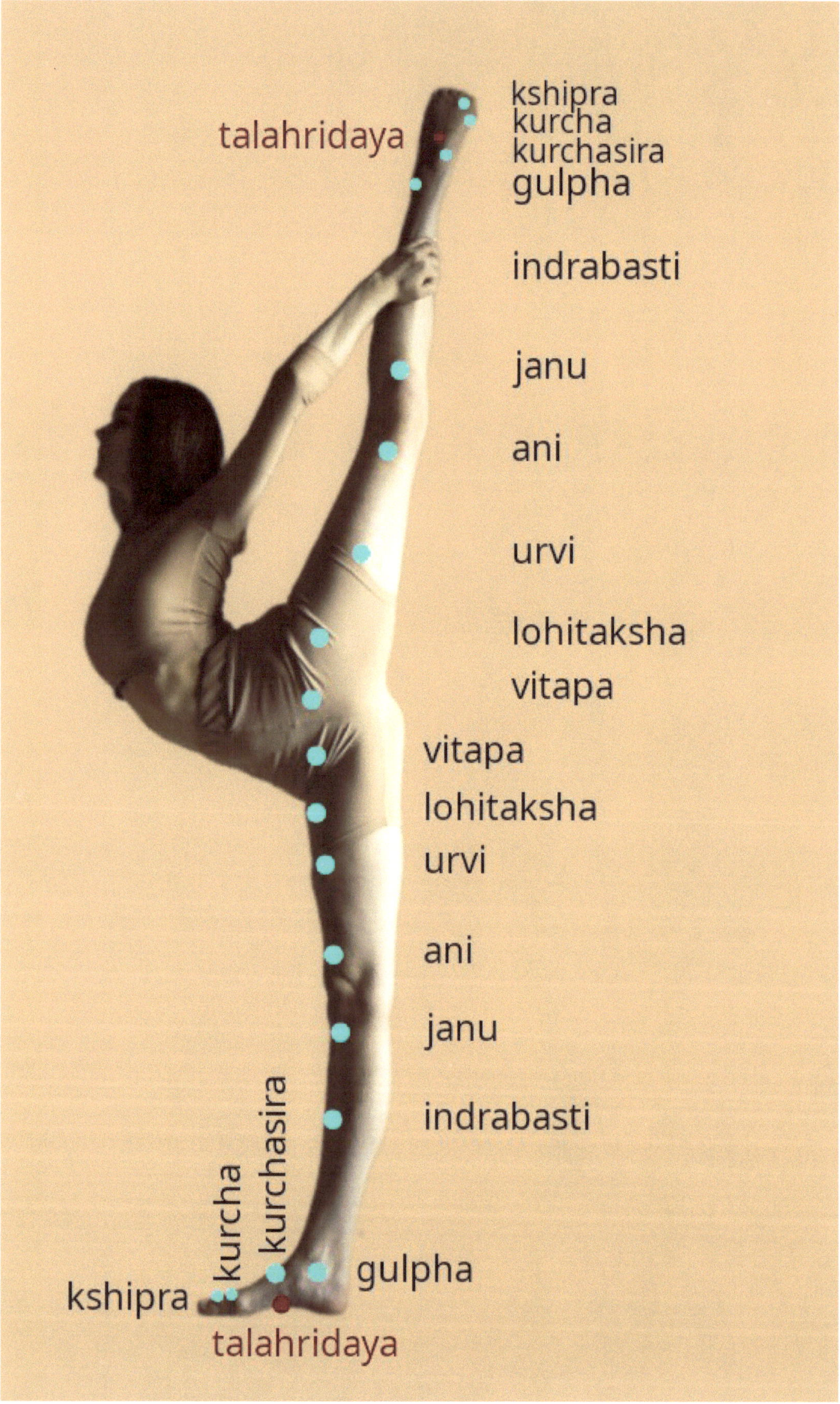

Figure 5 Marma Points in Leg and Foot (Side View)

Notes:
Kshipra is the point in between the big toe and adjacent toe.
Kurcha is at the base of big toe where it joins the foot, on top.
Talahridaya is on the sole of the foot, i.e., on bottom.

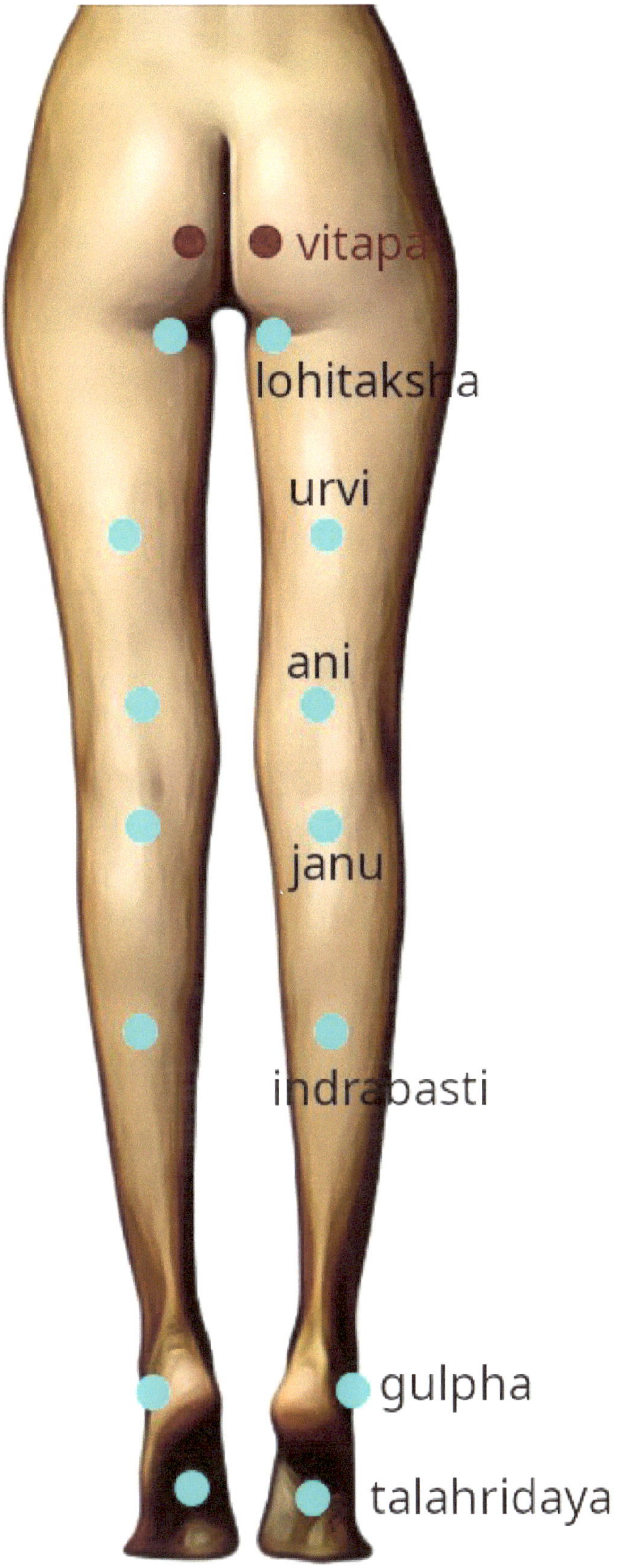

Figure 6 Marma Points in Legs and Feet (Posterior View)
Note: The Marma Points kūrcaśira, kūrca, kṣipra on feet are not visible in this diagram.
Note: Marma Points vitapa are shown in maroon since they are on the front side

Chest and Abdomen Marma Point Names

उदरोरसोस्तु गुदबस्तिनाभिहृदयस्तनमूलस्तनरोहितापलापान्यपस्तम्भौ चेति । Chest and Stomach marma points.

उदरः-उरसः-अस्तु गुद[1]-बस्ति[2]-नाभि[3]-हृदय[4]-स्तनमूल[5]-स्तनरोहित[6]-अपलापानि[7]-अपस्तम्भौ[8] चेति ।

- 8 apastambha (pair), *(topmost point in this list)* = vessel at side of breast containing vital air
- 7 apalāpa (pair) = cleavage that is ideally hidden
- 6 stanarohita (pair) = colored part of breast, above nipple
- 5 stanamūla (pair) = root of breast, below nipple
- 4 hṛdaya = heart
- 3 nābhi = navel
- 2 basti = bladder
- 1 guda *(bottommost point in this list)* = anus

A count of 12 points.

These points are listed in sequence of anatomical vertical location top to bottom.

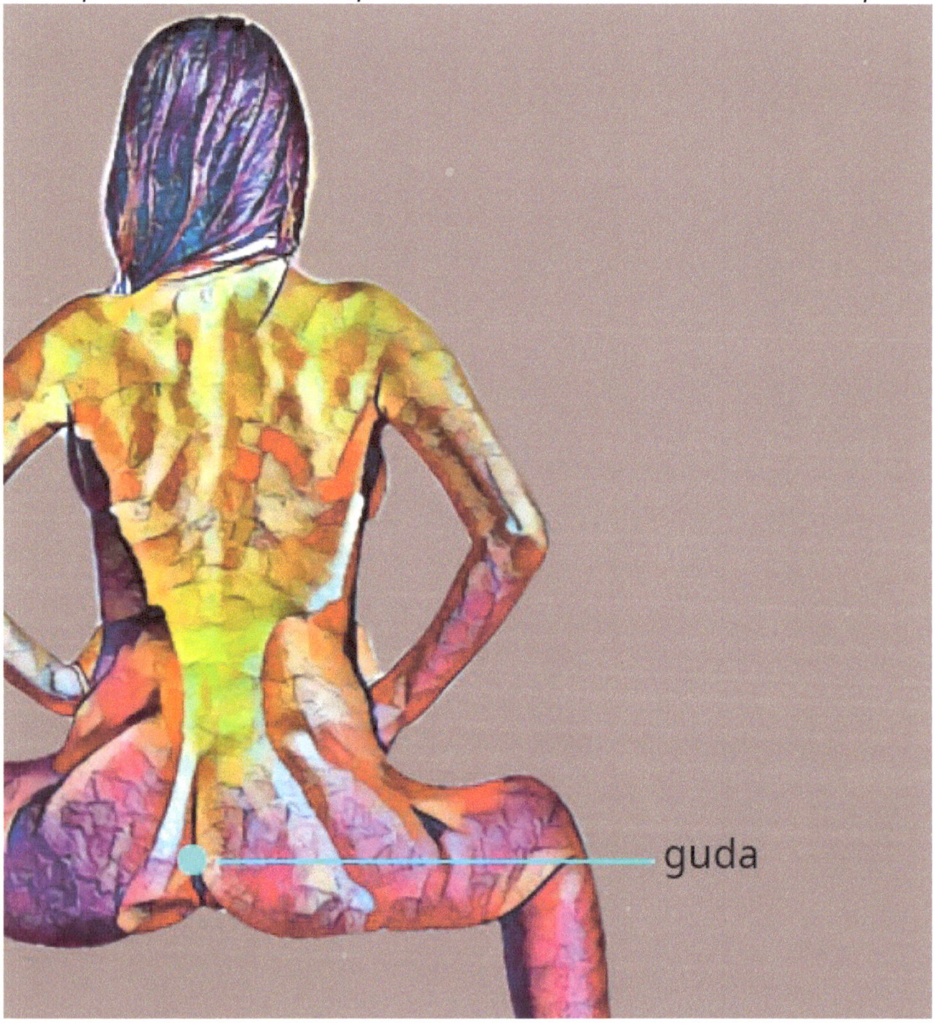

Figure 7 Marma Point Guda

Note: Even though Marma point guda is mentioned in "Chest and Abdomen", its exact location is at the place where the bums meet, the specific point which touches the seat when one is sitting. Hence it is behind on the backside as shown.

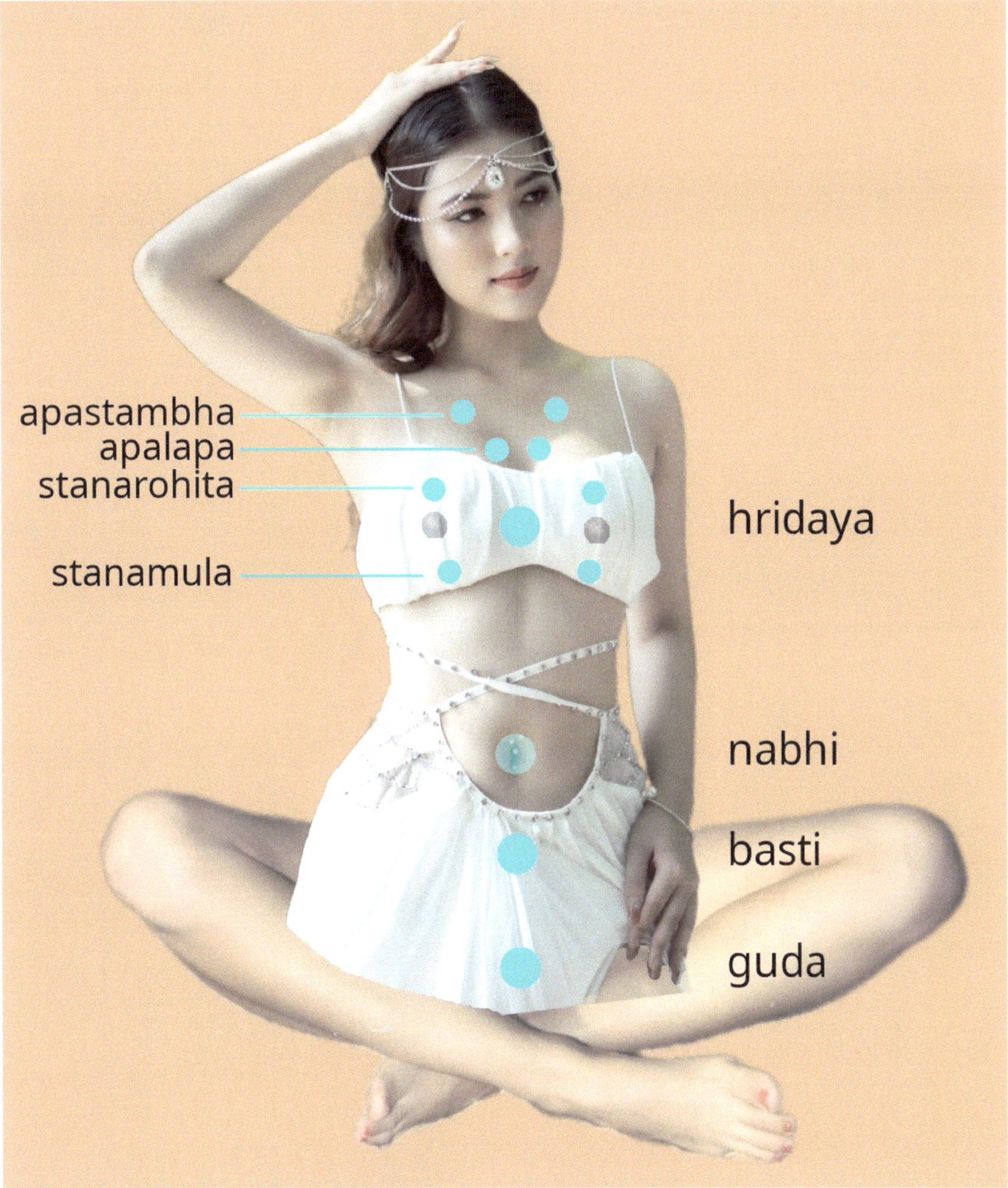

Figure 8 Marma Points in Chest and Abdomen

Note: Marma point guda is behind on the bums for therapy.

Back Marma Point Names (paired)

पृष्ठमर्माणि तु कटीकतरुणकुकुन्दरनितम्बपार्श्वसन्धिबृहत्यंसफलकान्यंसौ चेति । Marma Point names Behind, i.e. on the Back are listed.

पृष्ठ-मर्माणि तु कटीकतरुण[1]-कुकुन्दर[2]-नितम्ब[3]-पार्श्वसन्धि[4]-बृहती[5]-अंसफलकानि[6]-अंसौ[7] चेति ।

- 7 aṃsa (pair)
- 6 aṃsaphalaka (pair)
- 5 bṛhatī (pair)
- 4 pārśvasandhi (pair)
- 3 nitamba (pair)
- 2 kukundara (pair)
- 1 kaṭīkataruṇa (pair)

A count of 14 points.
These points are listed in sequence of anatomical vertical location top to bottom.

Notes on Marma Point Names
7 aṃsa अंस = Portion of shoulder right on top
6 aṃsaphalaka अंसफल = Extension of shoulder at back
5 bṛhatī बृहती = major middle Back area
4 pārśvasandhi पार्श्व-सन्धि = side Joints at back
3 nitamba नितम्ब = Hip
2 kukundara कुकुन्दर = V shape curve at edge of back, that houses organs for Digestive health
1 kaṭīkataruṇa कटीक-तरुण = veins very close to lowermost spine, those that keep us Youthful

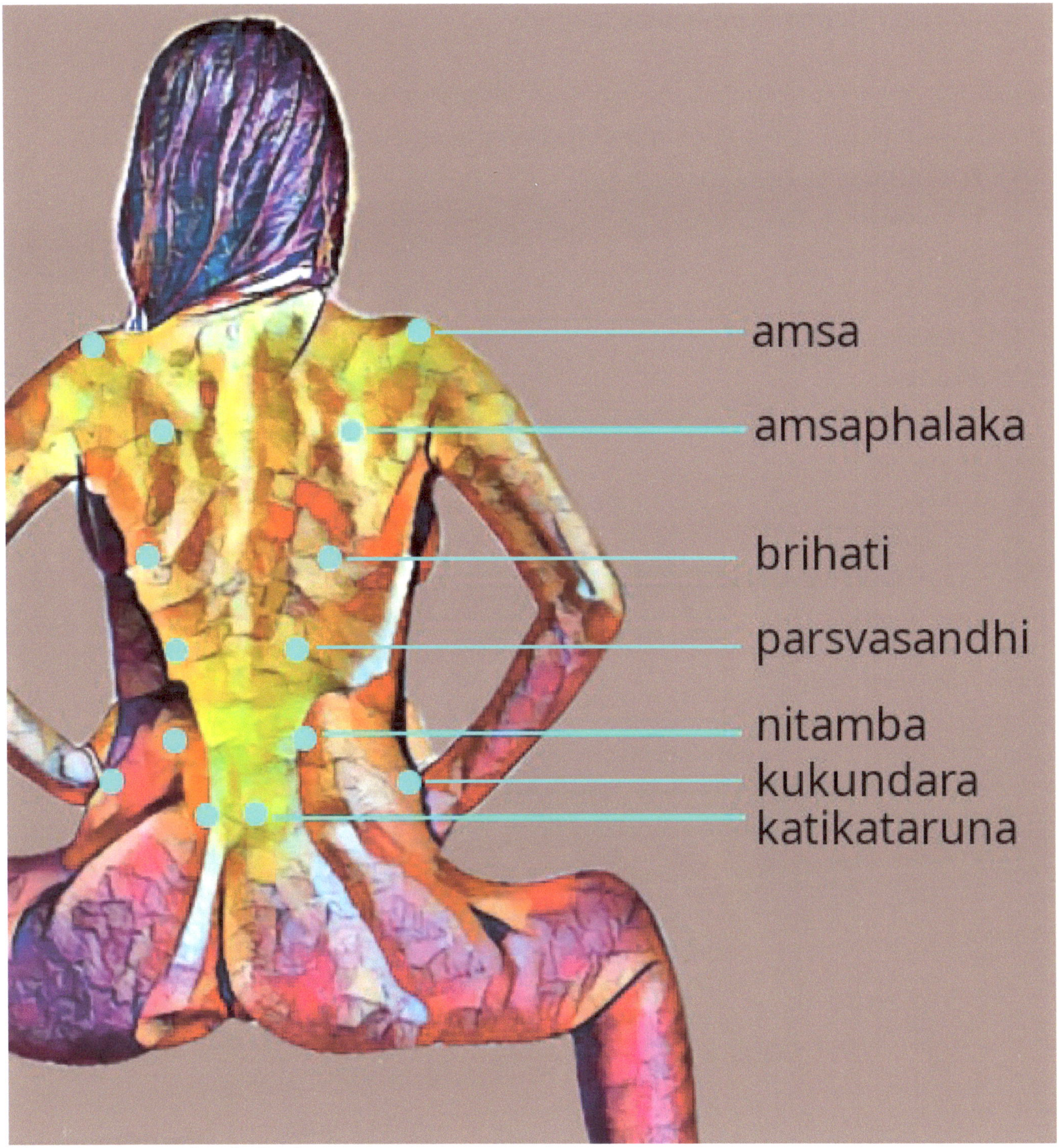

Figure 9 Marma Points in Back

Arm and Hand Marma Point Names (paired)

बाहुमर्माणि तु क्षिप्रतलहृदयकूर्चकूर्चशिरोमणिबन्धेन्द्रबस्तिकूर्पराण्युर्वीलोहिताक्षाणि कक्षधरं चेति । Arm Marma points list.
बाहु-मर्माणि तु क्षिप्र[1]-तलहृदय[2]-कूर्च[3]-कूर्चशिरः[4]-मणिबन्ध[5]-इन्द्रबस्ति[6]-कूर्पर[7]-आणि[8]-ऊर्वी[9]-लोहिताक्षाणि[10] कक्षधरं[11] चेति ।

- 11 kakṣadhara *(topmost point in this list)*
- 10 lohitākṣa
- 9 ūrvī
- 8 āṇi
- 7 kūrpara
- 6 indrabasti
- 5 maṇibandha
- 4 kūrcaśira
- 3 kūrca
- 2 talahṛdaya
- 1 kṣipra *(bottommost point in this list)*

These points are listed in sequence of vertical location top to bottom of anatomy.
Note: The Marma points **Kakṣadhara**, **Kūrpara** and **Maṇibandha** in **arm** correspond to **Viṭapa**, **Jānu** and **Gulpha** in **leg** respectively.

एतेनेतरो बाहुर्व्याख्यातः । These are **mirrored** in each arm, so a count of 22 points.

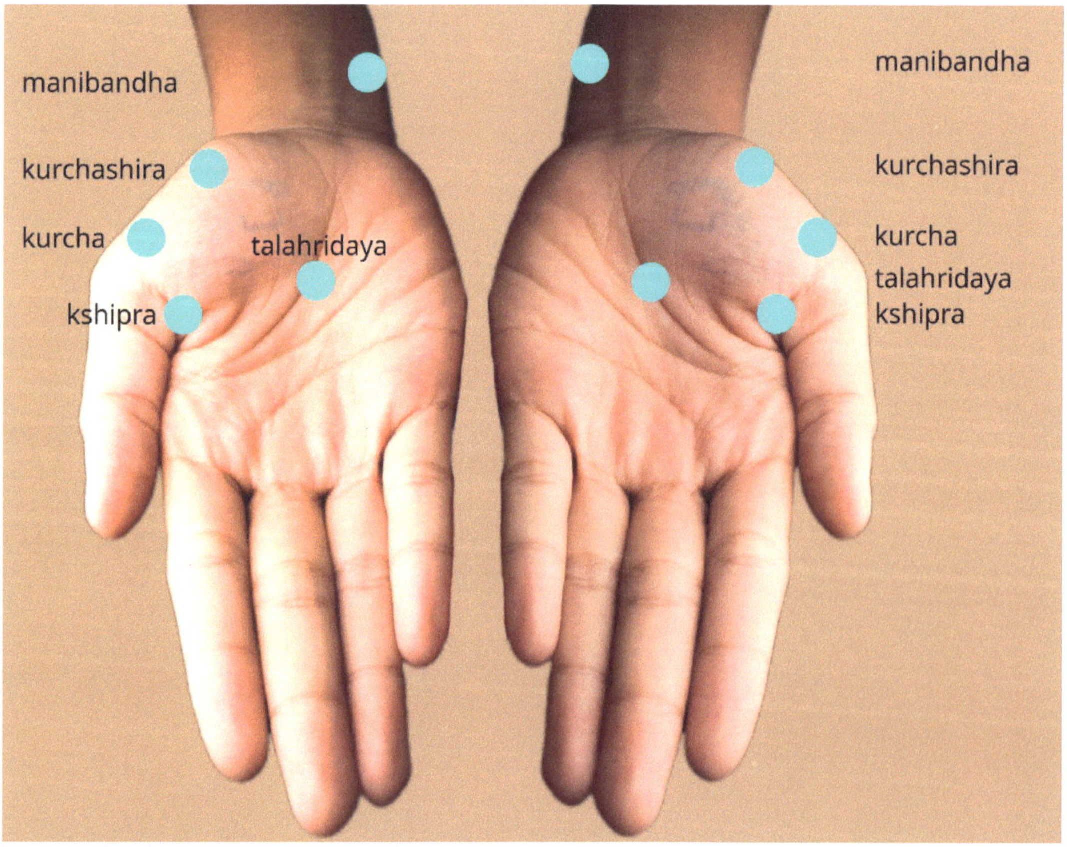

Figure 10 Marma Points in Hands

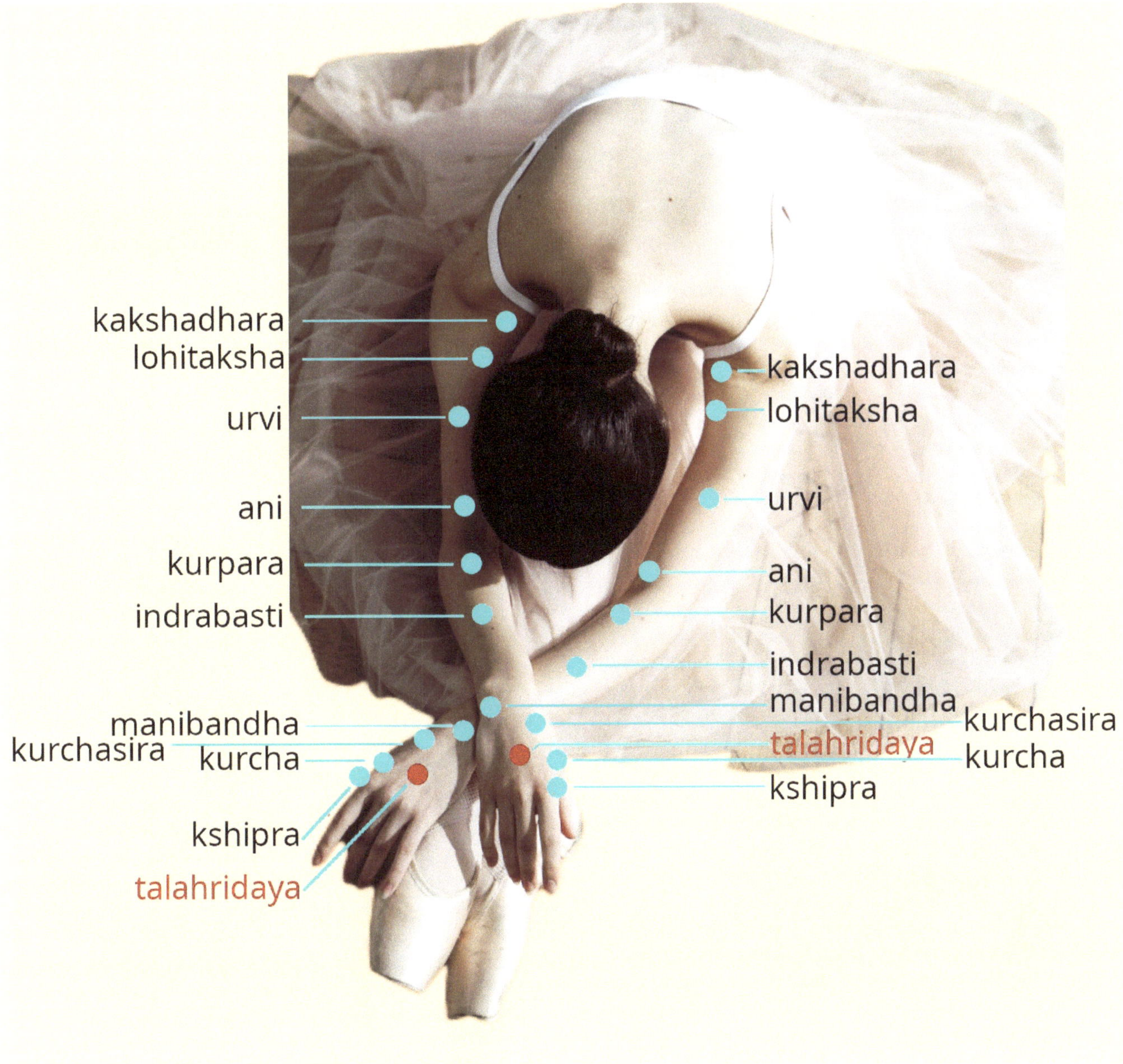

Figure 11 Marma Points in Arms and Hands

Note: Talahridaya is in the **palm** and not at the back of the hand.

6 indrabasti is located at the approximate **center** of **forearm**.

5 maṇibandha is located just **below** the **wrist bone**. (*reflection of* ***gulpha*** *at foot*).

4 kūrcaśira is located at the **junction endpoint** of thumb and wrist.

3 kūrca is located at the **far extremity** of the **thumb** where it joins the hand.

2 talahṛdaya is located at the approximate **center** of **palm**.

1 kśipra is located at the **junction** of **thumb and index finger**, where these join the palm.

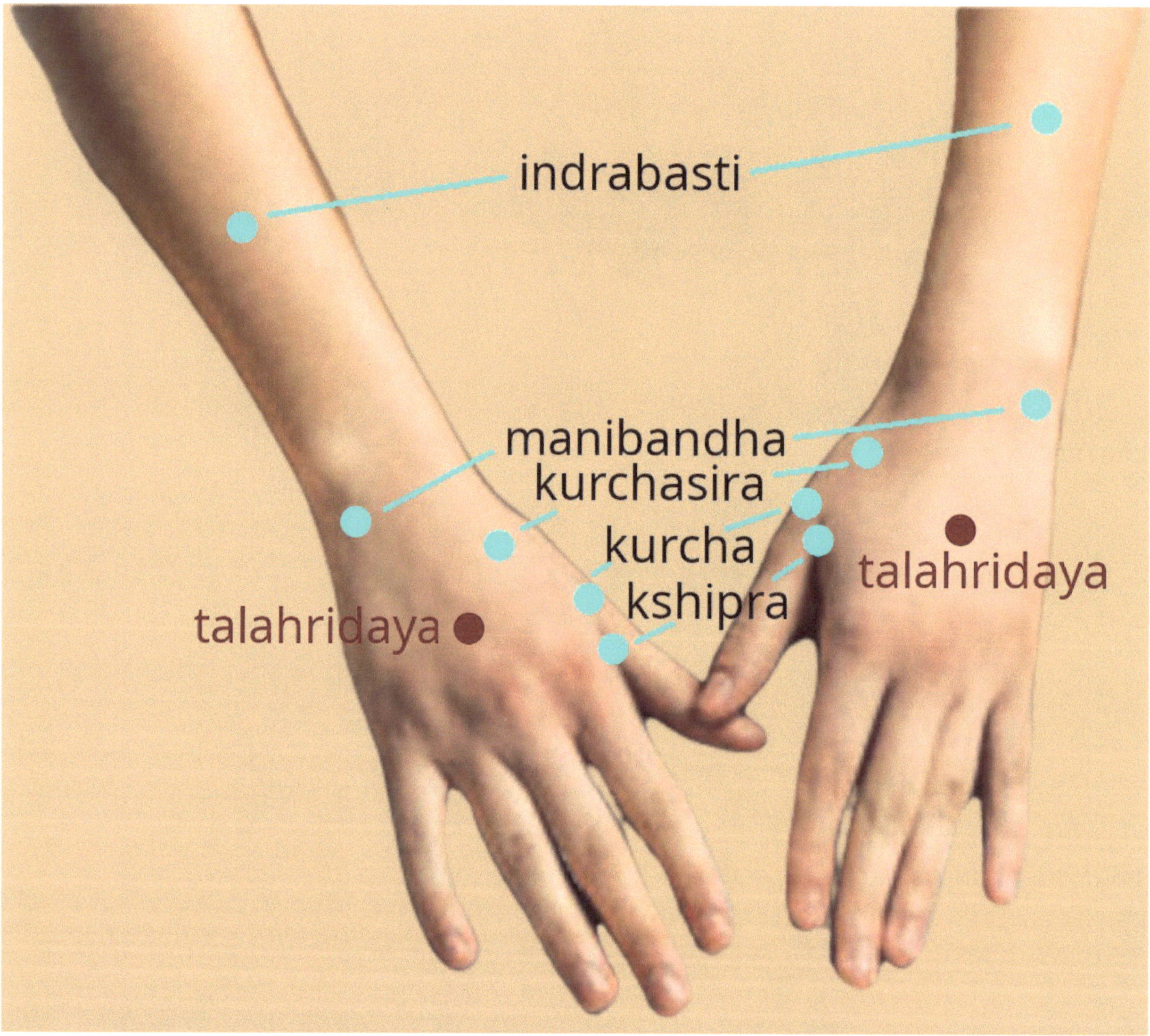

Figure 12 Marma Points in Hands

Note: Talahridaya is in the **palm** and not at the back of the hand.

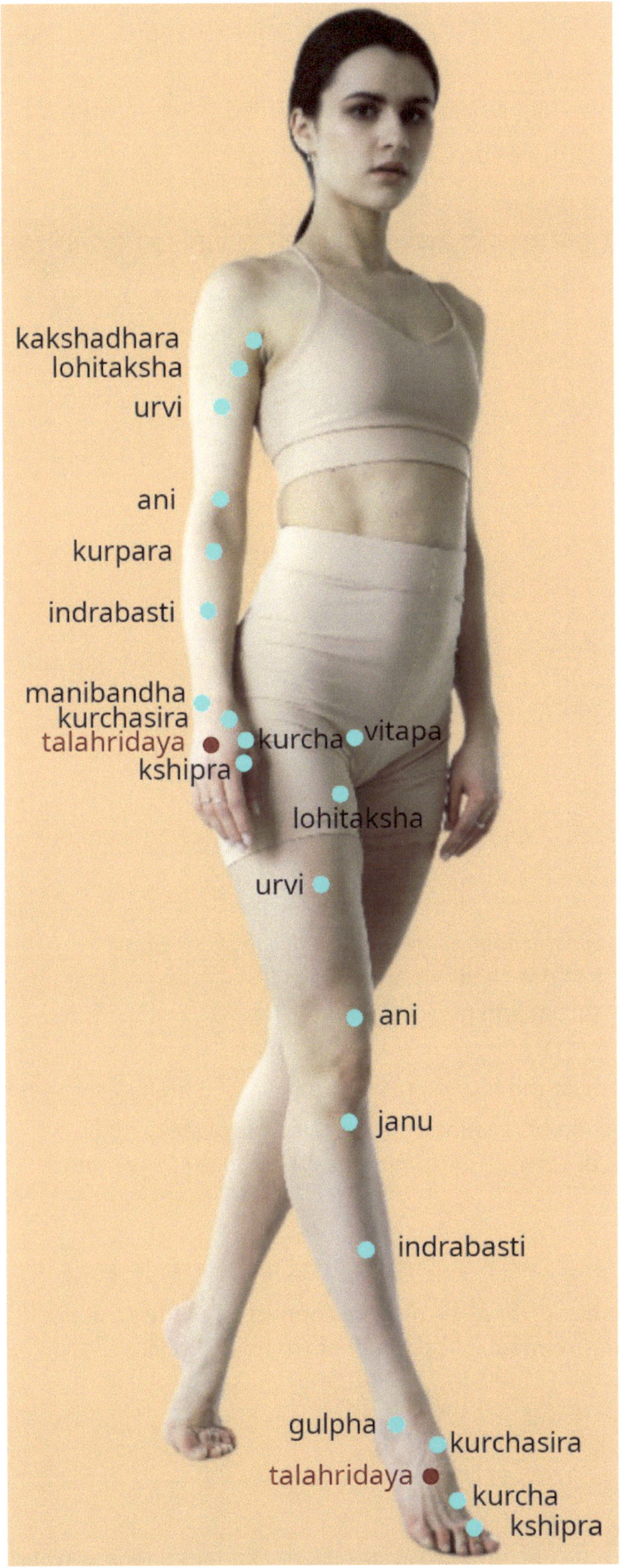

Figure 13 Marma Points in Arms wrt Feet

Head and Neck Marma Point Names

जत्रुण ऊर्ध्वं चतस्रो धमन्योऽष्टौ मातृका द्वे कृकाटिके द्वे विधुरे द्वे फणे द्वावपाङ्गौ द्वावावर्तौ द्वावुत्क्षेपौ द्वौ शङ्खावेका स्थपनी पञ्च सीमन्ताश्च त्वारि शृङ्गाटकान्येकोऽधिपतिरिति ॥ ७ ॥ Marma Point names **Above the Clavicle** are listed.

जत्रुण ऊर्ध्वं चतस्रो धमनि[1]-अष्टौ मातृका[2] द्वे कृकाटिके[3] द्वे विधुरे[4] द्वे फणे[5] द्वावपाङ्गौ[6] द्वावावर्तौ[7] द्वावुत्क्षेपौ[8] द्वौ शङ्खौ[9] एका स्थपनी[10] पञ्च सीमन्ताः[11] चत्वारि शृङ्गाटकानि[12] एक अधिपतिः[13] इति ॥

- 13 adhipati *(topmost point in this list)*
- 12 śṛṅgāṭaka (four)
- 11 sīmanta (five)
- 10 sthapanī
- 9 śaṅkha (pair)
- 8 utkṣepa (pair)
- 7 āvarta (pair)
- 6 apāṅga (pair)
- 5 phaṇa (pair)
- 4 vidhura (pair)
- 3 kṛkāṭikā (pair)
- 2 mātṛkā (eight)
- 1 dhamani (four), *(bottommost point in this list)*

A count of 37 points. *Here **not** all points are in sequence of anatomical vertical location top to bottom.*

Marma Points adhipati, sīmanta are on the head.
Marma Points śṛṅgāṭaka, sthapanī, śaṅkhā, utkṣepa, āvarta, apāṅga, phaṇa are in the face region.
Marma Points vidhura, kṛkāṭikā, and some mātṛkā are in the neck region at rear.
Marma Points mātṛkā some, and dhamani are in the throat and neck region at front.

The Marma Point धमनि = नीला + मन्या **dhamani** consists of the four points named **nīlā** and **manyā** pairs, as clarified in verses 8, 14, 27. Here **nīlā** refers to points on **blue veins** on either side of trachea, while **manyā** refers to points on **red arteries** on either side of trachea. (*Alternate name for **manyā** is **mantha.** Alternate name for **nīlā** is **sirāmantha***).

The Marma Point मातृका = कण्ठ + कण्ठनाडी + अक्षक at front, + ग्रीवा + मन्यामानि + पृष्ठग्रीवा at back = **mātṛkā** consists of eight points on four pairs on *tubes* on either side of neck, directly connected to the nose and throat. These points are *technically* named **kaṇṭha, kaṇṭhanādī, akṣaka pair** at frontside, **grīvā, manyāmani, pṛṣṭhagrīvā pair** at backside.
Note: mātṛkā consists of eight points, four at front and four at back of neck.
grīvā = reflection of kaṇṭha on top of neck at backside.
manyāmani = reflection of kaṇṭhanādī on base of neck at backside.
pṛṣṭhagrīvā pair = reflection of akṣaka pair at base of neck at backside.

- Marma pairs **nīlā, manyā** and **akṣaka** are technically located on the sternocleidomastoid muscle.
- Marma point **kaṇṭha** is located at the junction center of neck with head.
- Marma point **kaṇṭhanādī** is located in the groove below adam's apple.

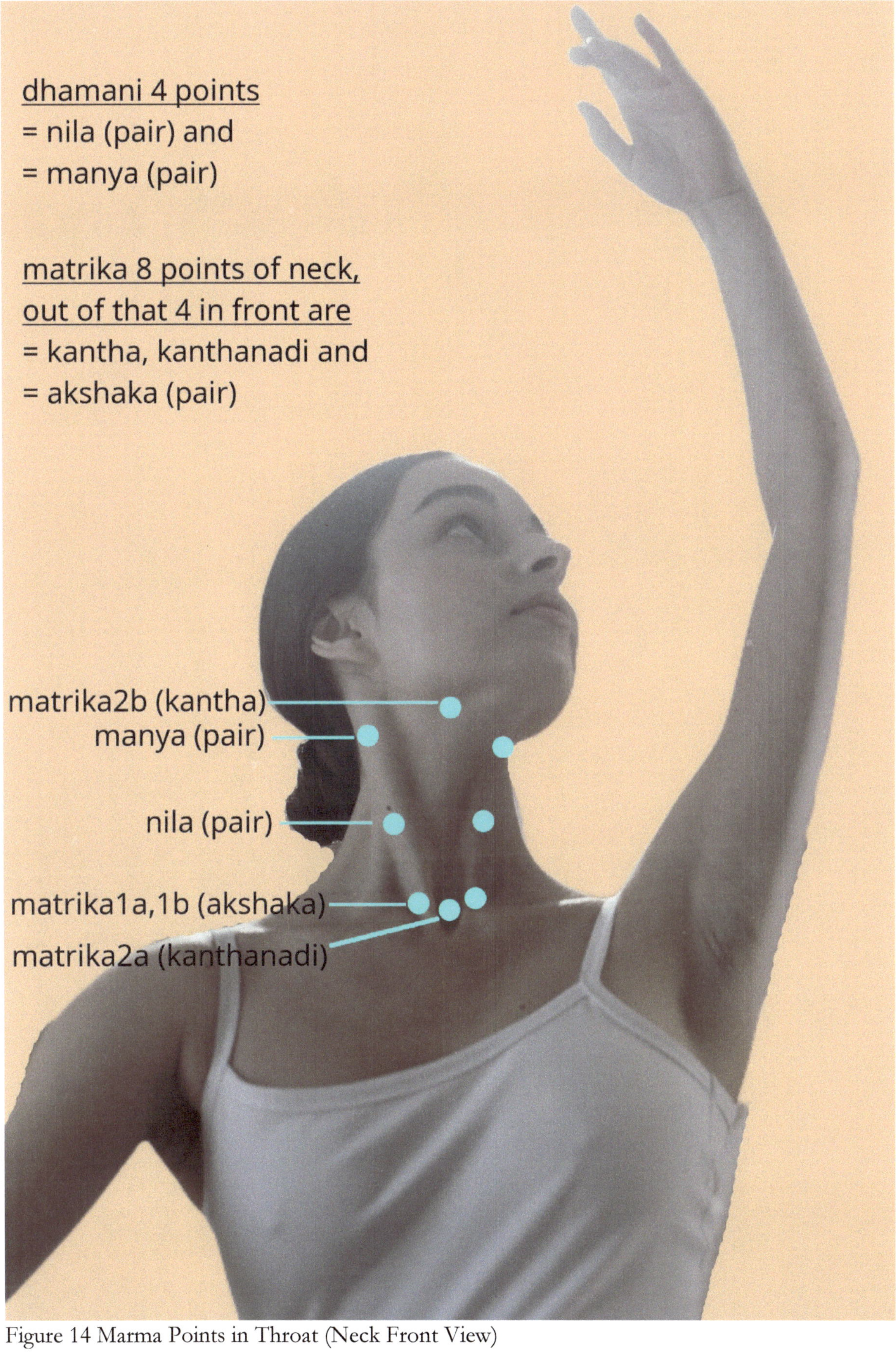

Figure 14 Marma Points in Throat (Neck Front View)

Note: Only four matrika points seen here out of eight. Rest four are at back of Neck.
All four Dhamani Points are seen. Nila (pair) and Manya (pair).

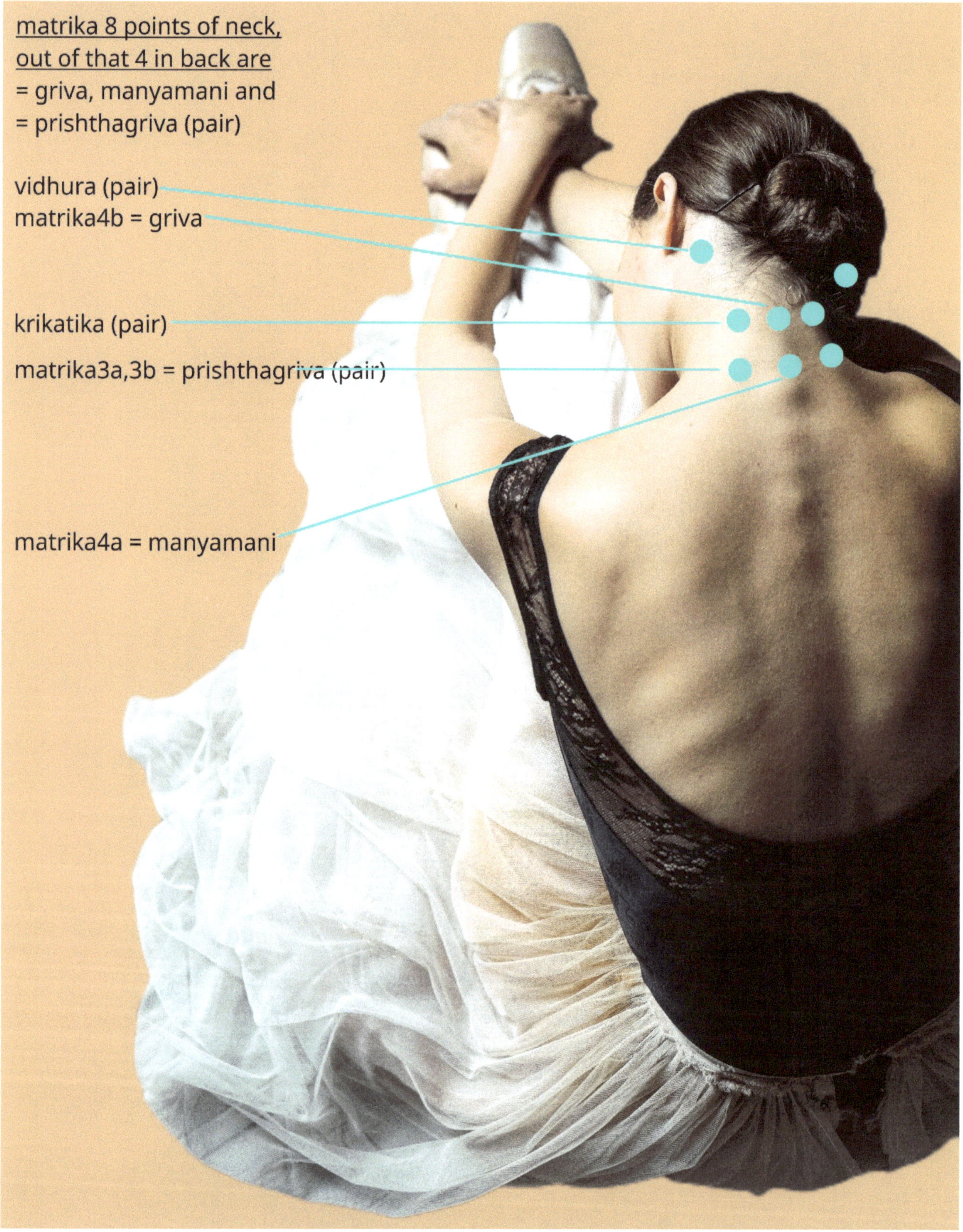

Figure 15 Marma Points in Neck (Rear View)

Note: Only four matrika points seen here out of eight.

Matrika points at back = Prishtagriva pair, Manyamani, Griva

Other points on neck rear are Vidhura (pair), and Krikatika (pair)

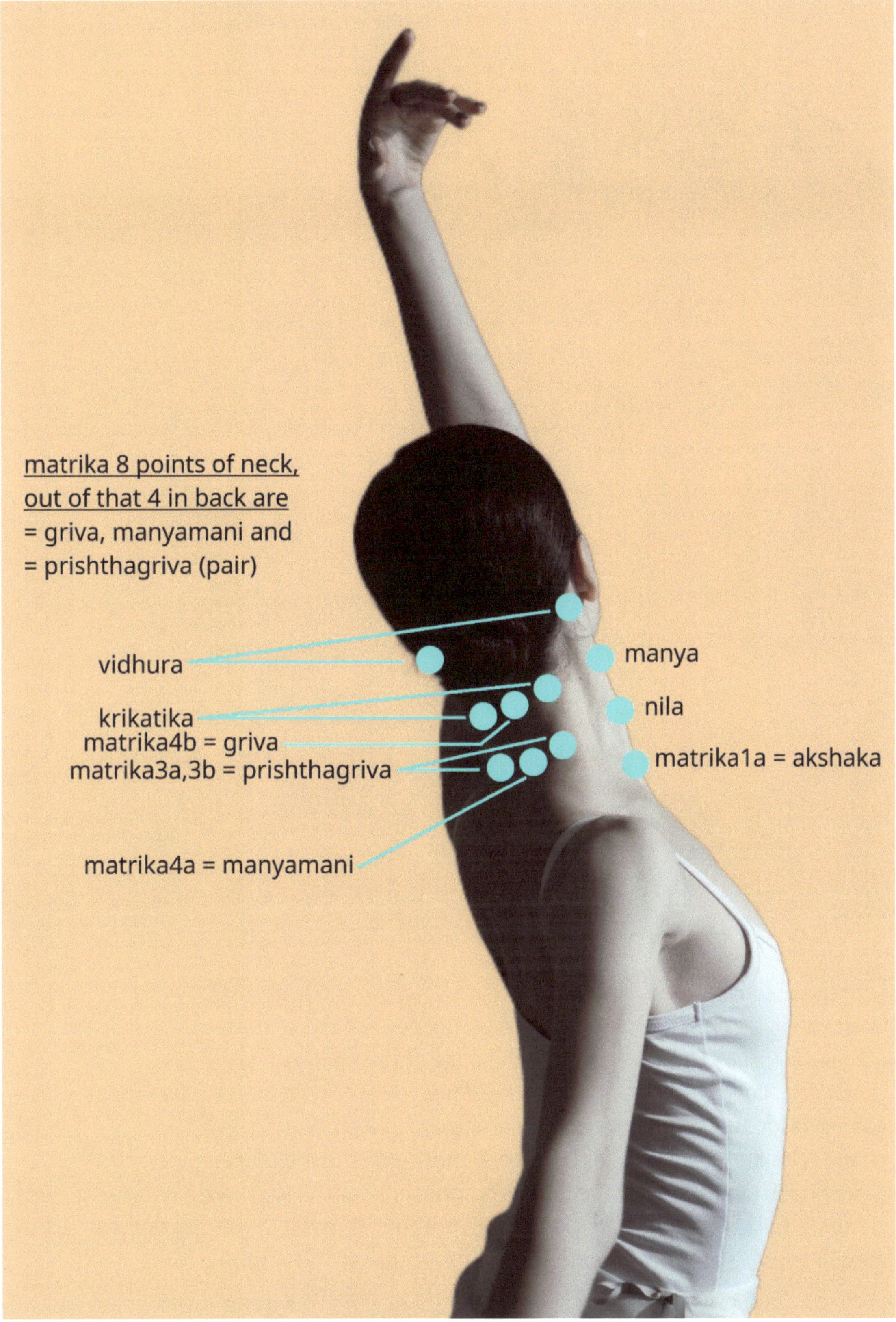

Figure 16 Marma Points in Neck (Side View)

Visible Matrika 4 points at back = griva, manyamani, prishthagriva (pair)
Matrika 1 of 4 points at front = akshaka (mirrored pair is not in view, kantha, kanthanadi not in view)
Dhamani 2 of 4 points at front = nila, manya (mirrored pair is not in view)

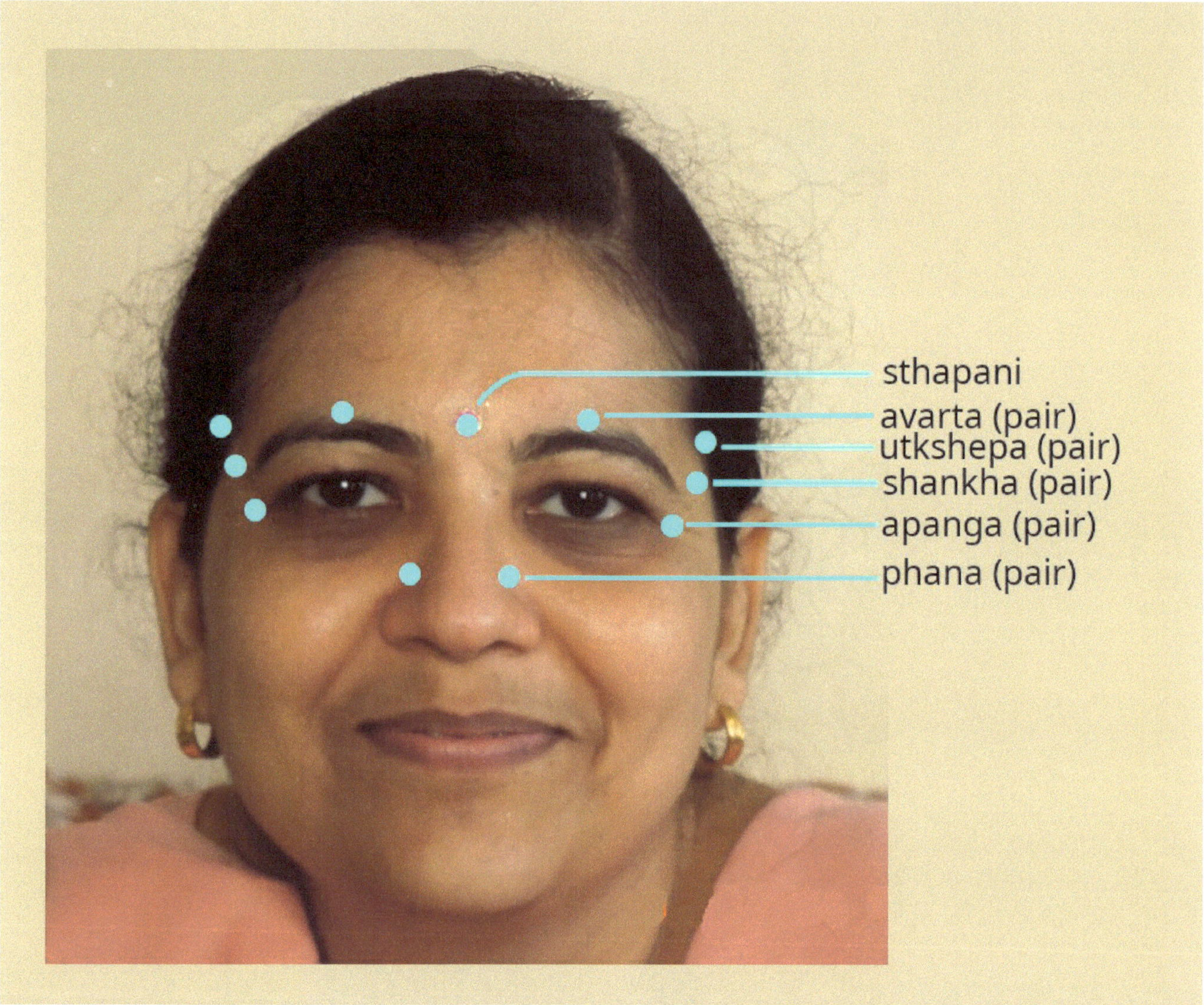

Figure 17 Marma Points in Face except shringataka

Notes:

- Marma point **sthapanī** is located on the ajna chakra in between the eyebrows.
- Marma pair **āvarta** is located above the eye center at the edge of the eyebrow.
- Marma pair **utkṣepa** is located above śaṅkhā at the edge of the hairline in a groove.
- Marma pair **śaṅkhā** is located on the temples in a groove.
- Marma pair **apāṅga** is located on the outer edge of the eye in a groove.
- Marma pair **phaṇa** is located on the outer edges of the nose on the maxillary sinus.
- Marma points **śṛṅgāṭaka** are related to the nerves responsible for the four sense organs viz. eyes, ears, nose, and tongue. Though mentioned as four in number, in practice we classify them as
  - 1 Related to Eyes pupil **कनीनका kanīnakā** pair**,** eyebrow **भ्रू अन्तरा bhrū antarā**,
  - 2 Related to Ears top **कर्णपाल karṇapāla** pair, ear lobes **कर्णपालि karṇapāli** pair
  - 3 Related to Nose at cheek **कपोल नासा kapola nāsā** pair, nosetip **नासापुट nāsāpuṭa**
  - 4 Related to Tongue **ओष्ठ oṣṭha** one, **हनु hanu** one, **कपोल मध्यमा kapola madhyamā** pair

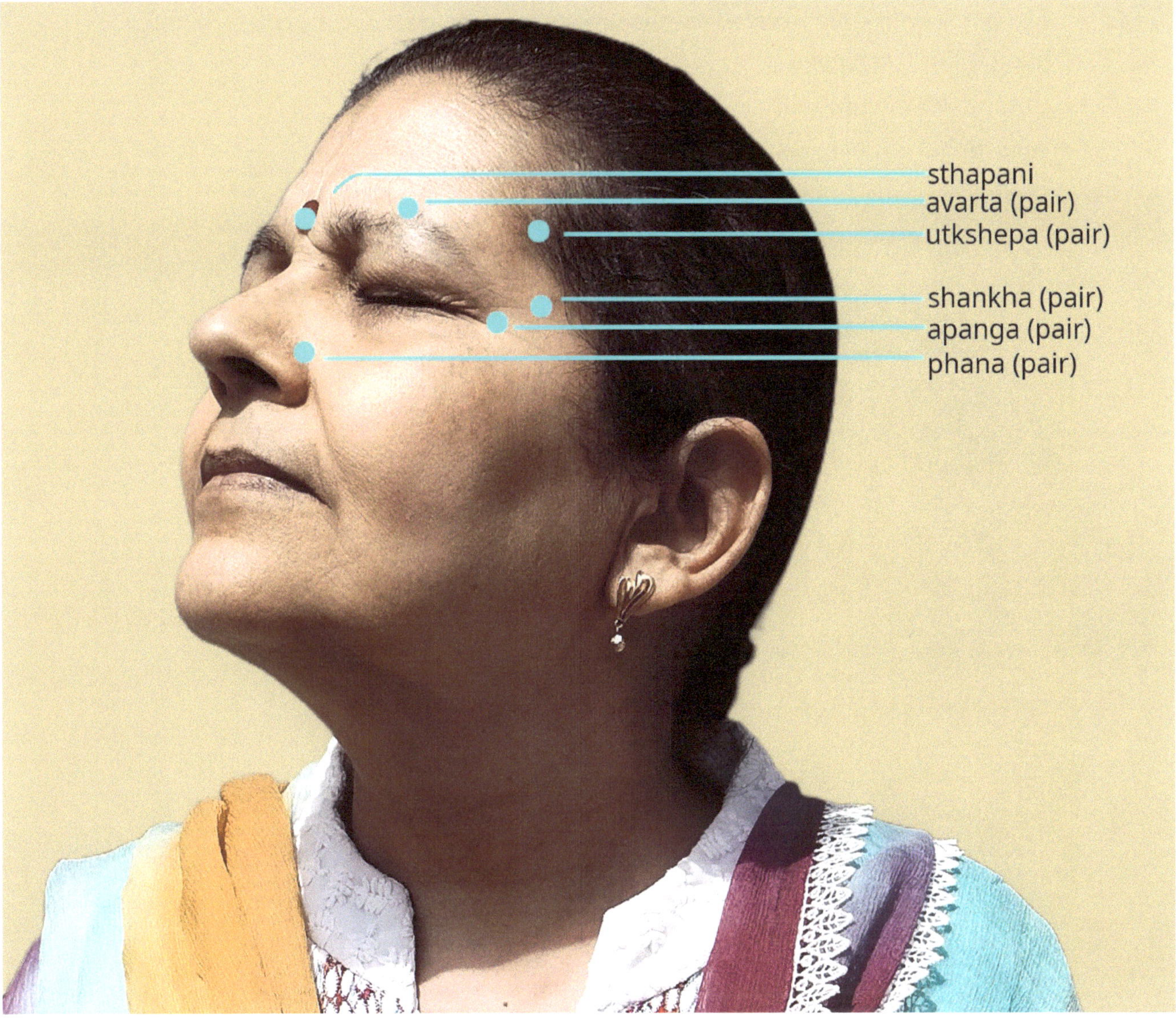

Figure 18 Marma Points in Face (Side View) except shringataka

Marma points **śṛṅgāṭaka** on nerves related to four sense organs as stated in Sushruta Samhita

- Eyes: pupil कनीनका **kanīnakā**
- Ears: earlobe कर्णपालि **karṇapāli**
- Nose: nose tip कपोलनासा **kapolanāsā**
- Tongue: lip ओष्ठ **oṣṭha** and chin हनु **hanu**

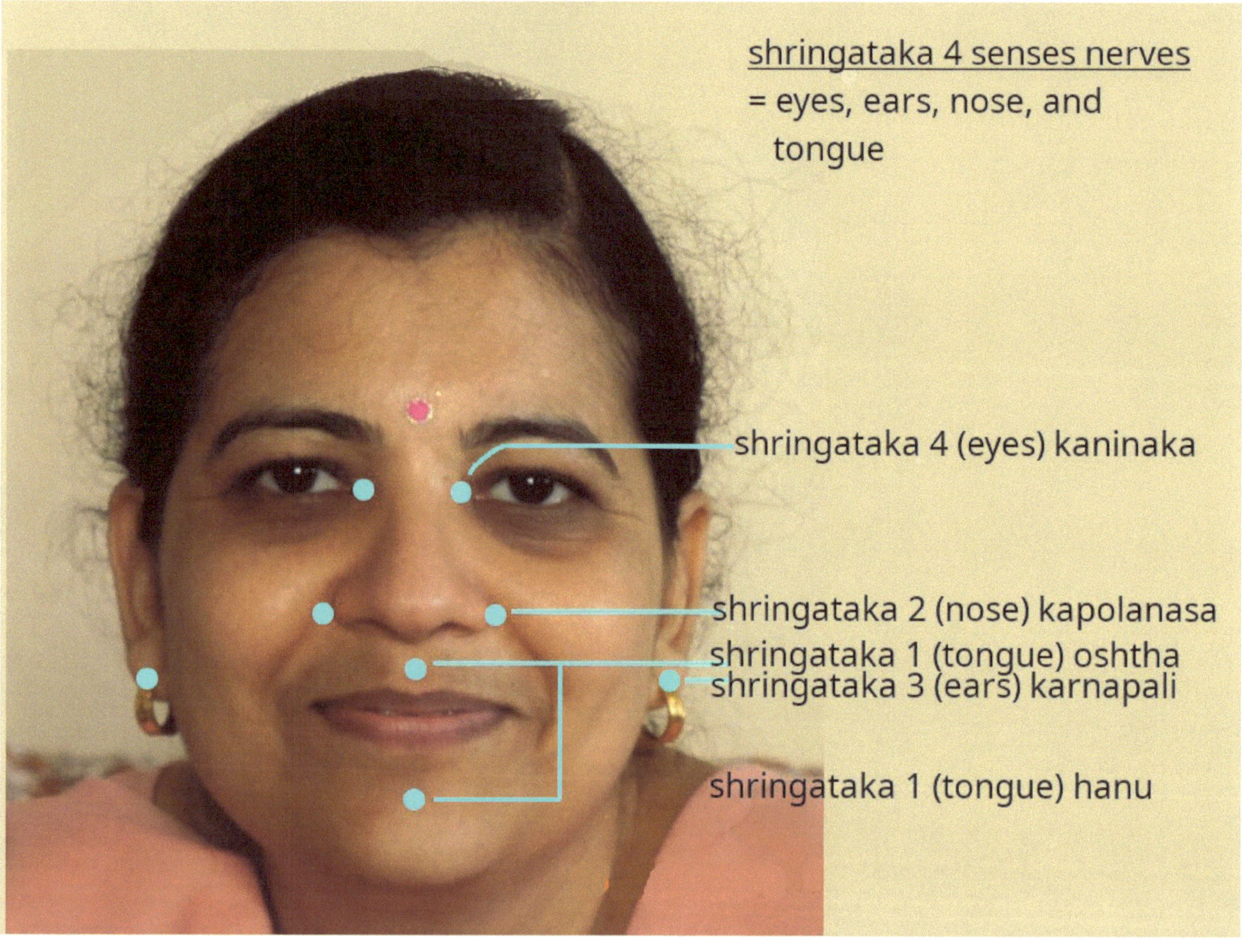

Figure 19 Marma Points Shringataka on 4 Sense Organ Nerves

Note: As per the Samhita there are 4 points in all, however in practice we take 4 pairs.

Shringataka 4 Related to Eyes - pupil कनीनका **kanīnakā** pair

Shringataka 3 Related to Ears - ear lobes कर्णपालि **karṇapāli** pair

Shringataka 2 Related to Nose - at cheek कपोल नासा **kapola nāsā** pair

Shringataka 1 Related to Tongue ओष्ठ **oṣṭha** one, हनु **hanu** one

Marma points **śṛṅgāṭaka** on nerves related to four sense organs as used in Marma Chikitsa Practice

- Eyes:
    - eyebrow inner edge भ्रू अन्तरा **bhrū antarā** pair
    - pupil कनीनका **kanīnakā** pair
    - lower eyelid palpebra मध्य वर्त्म **madhya vartma** pair
- Ears:
    - top of ear कर्णपाल **karṇapāla** pair
    - bottom earring point कर्णपालि **karṇapāli** pair
- Nose:
    - nostril extremity कपोल नासा **kapola nāsā** pair
    - nose tip नासापुट **nāsāpuṭa**
- Tongue:
    - lip ओष्ठ **oṣṭha**
    - jaw कपोल मध्यमा **kapola madhyamā** pair
    - chin हनु **hanu**

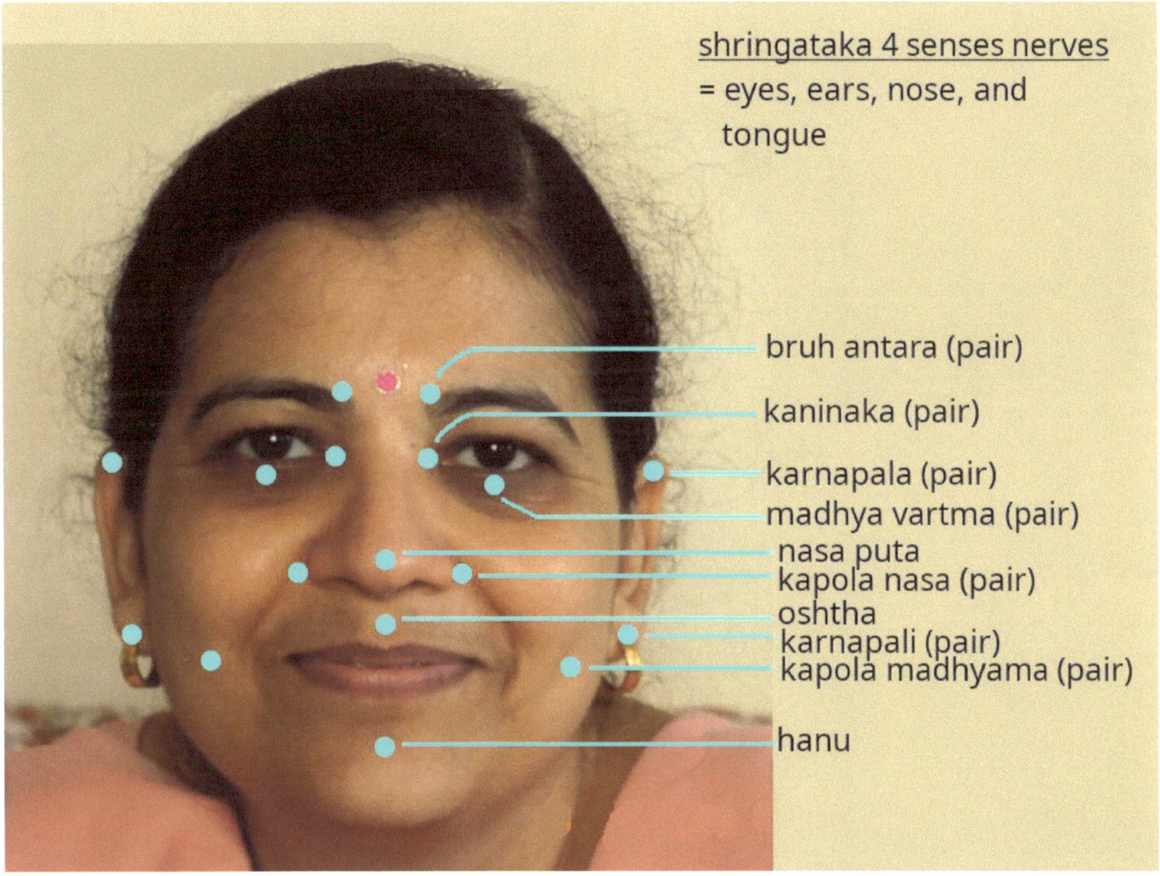

Figure 20 Marma Points Shringataka on 4 Sense Organ Nerves in Practice

Marma points on **Face** from Head and Neck as in **Marma Chikitsa Practice**

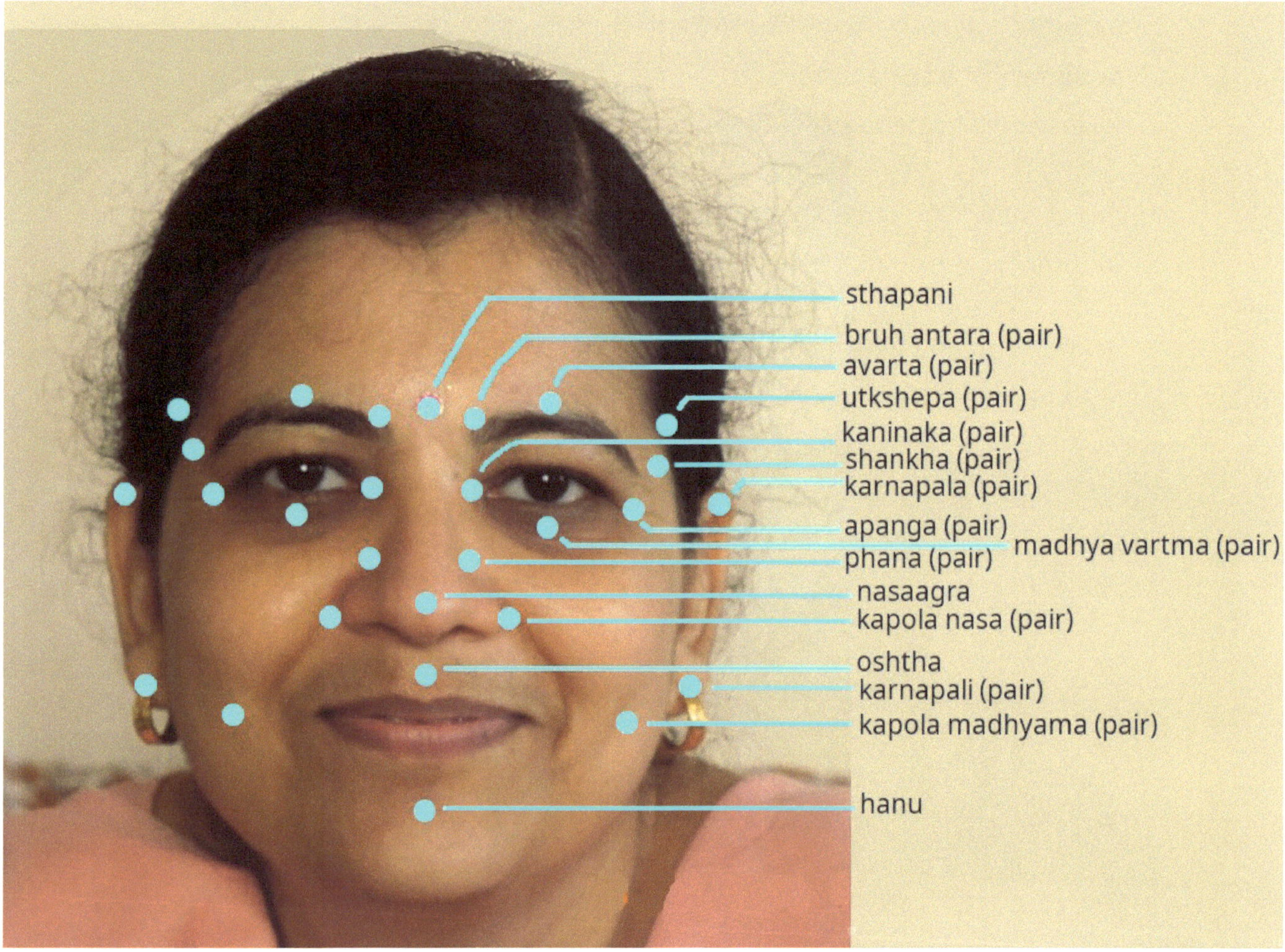

Figure 21 Marma Points on Face in Practice

Marma points on **Skull** from Head and Neck

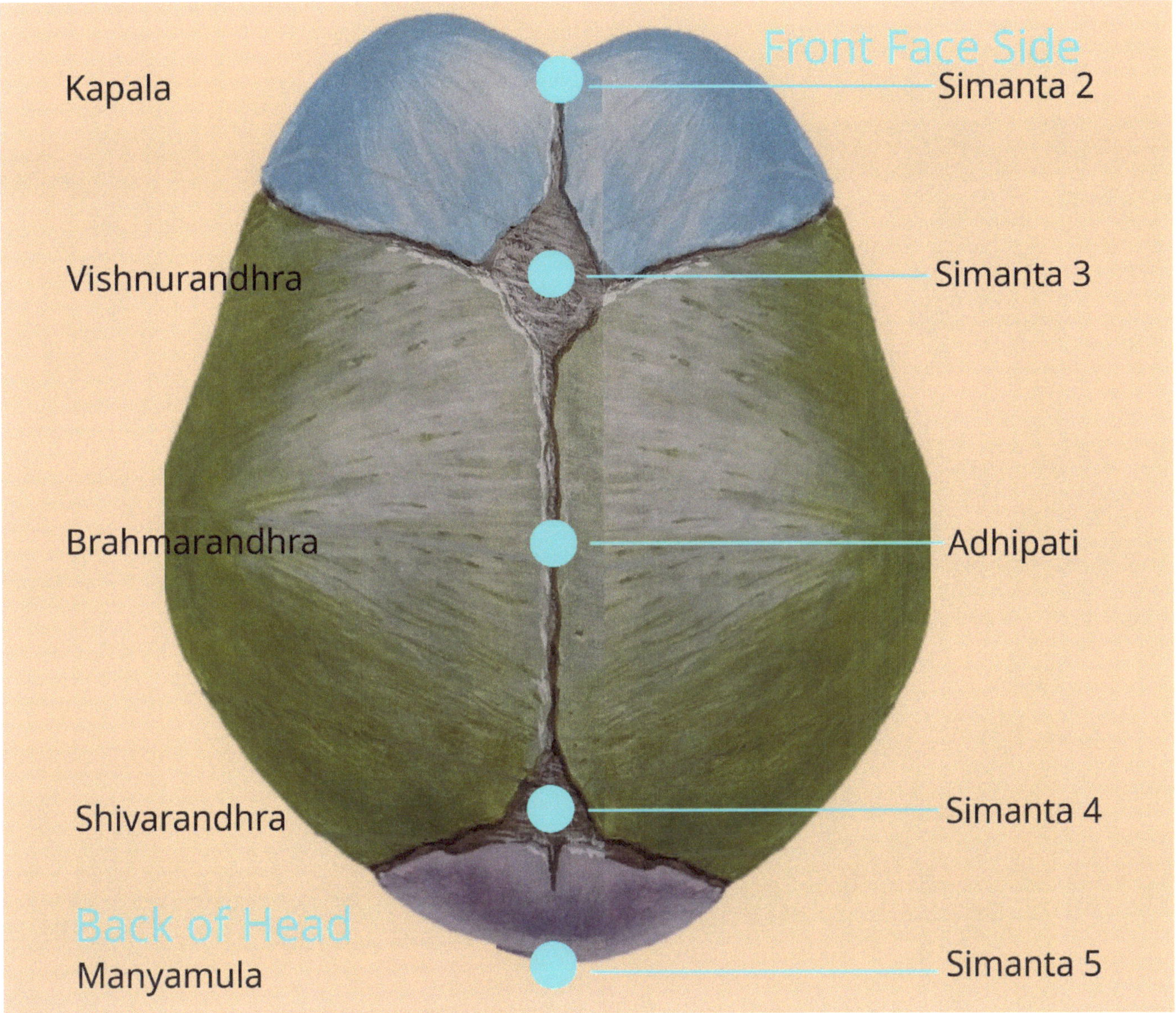

Figure 22 Marma Points on Skull (Top View)

Note: Position of Simanta1 and Simanta2 is clear in another diagram showing front of head.
Note: Position of Simanta5 is clear in another diagram showing back of head.
Note: The term Brahmarandhra is frequently seen in literature, called the crown or sahasrara chakra. However, for the case of Marma, this 7th chakra or sahasrara is split as the two points viz. Simanta3 (Vishnurandhra) and Adhipati (Brahmarandhra).

Another point Simanta4 (Shivarandhra) is the point where there is a tuft of hair, and girls tie a pony tail, called शिखा **Śikhā** in Sanskrit.

Marma points on **Skull** from Head and Neck as in **Marma Chikitsa Practice**

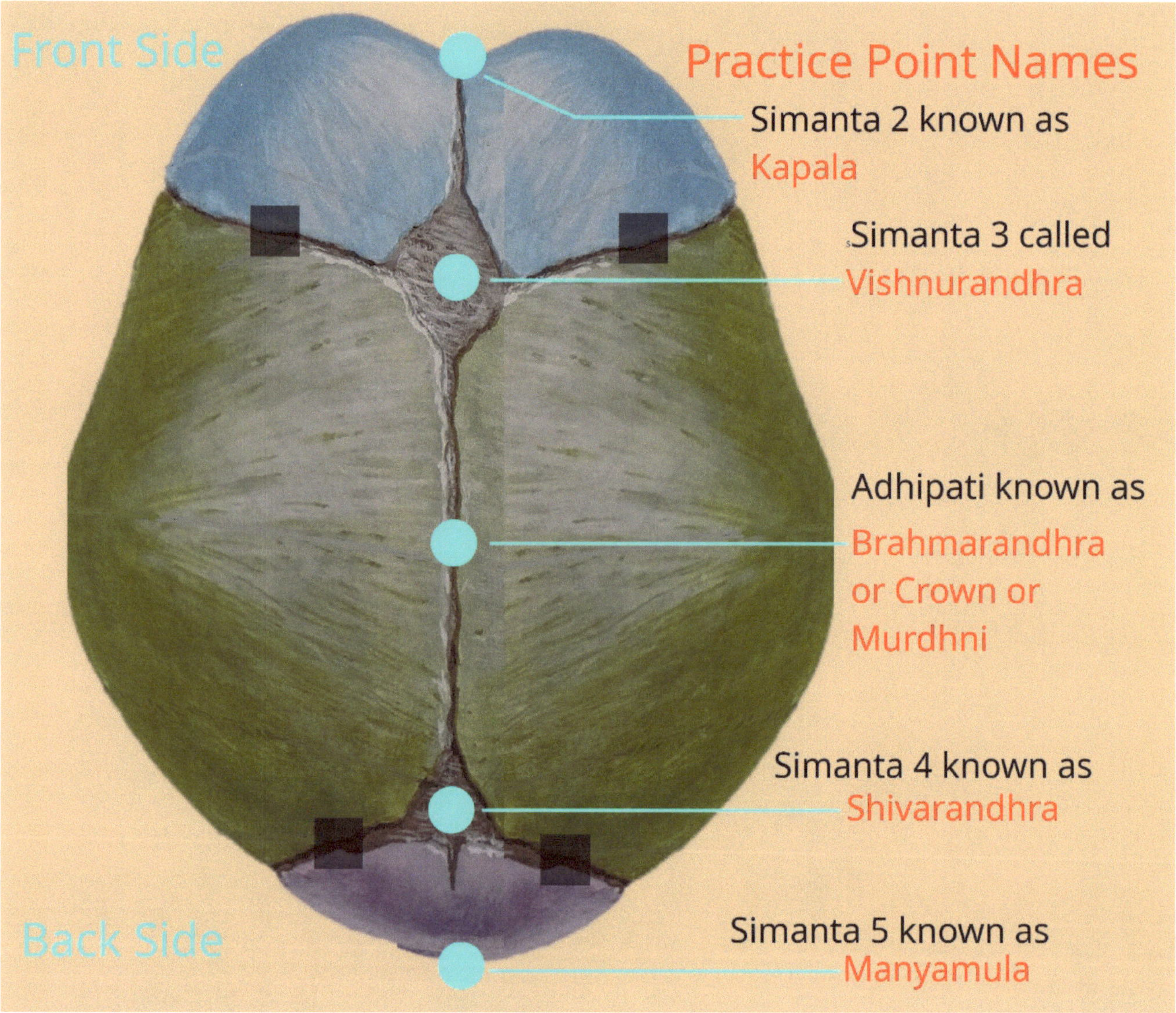

Figure 23 Marma Practice Points on Skull (Top View)

Note: Simanta1 is not visible here
Note: For Marma Chikitsa Therapy, the Simanta points are named as given and pressed accordingly.
Note: The terms Vishnurandhra and Brahmarandhra are sometimes used interchangeably.
Note: **Charaka** Samhita uses the term **Murdhni** (for Adhipati of Sushruta Samhita).

Note: The Marma Points Simanta are five in number, and literally सीमन्त means the edges and extremities of the skull, in a line.

Marma points on **Skull** from Side as in **Marma Chikitsa Practice**

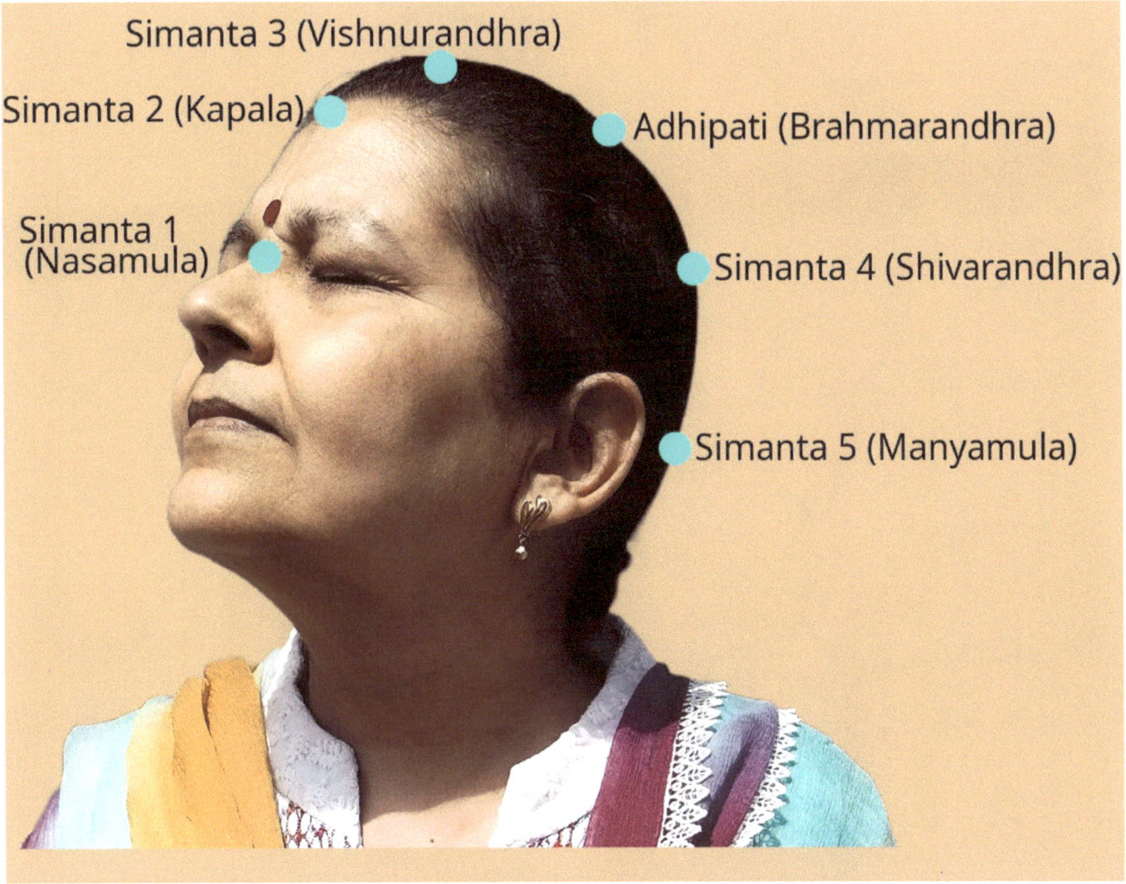

Figure 24 Marma Points Simanta five nos and Adhipati (Left Side View)

Figure 25 Marma Points Simanta and Adhipati (Right Side View)

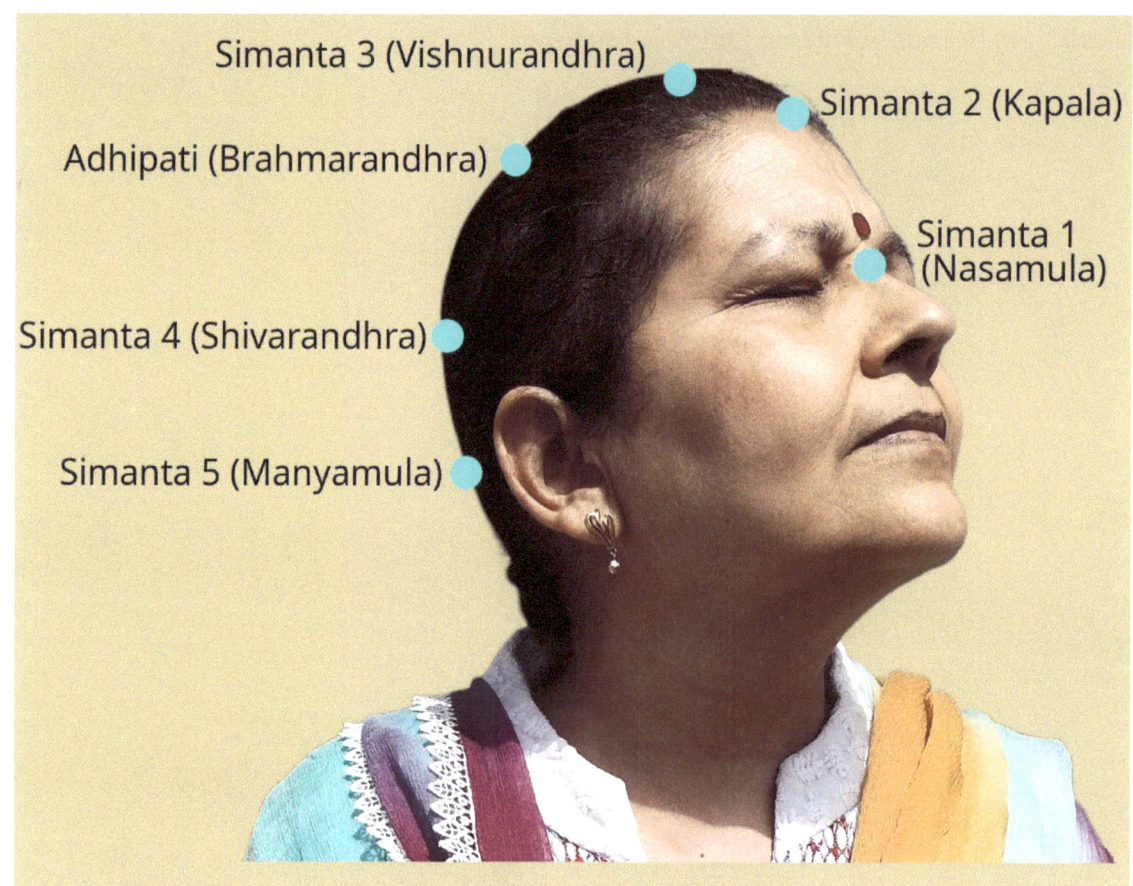

Marma points on **Skull** from Head and Neck as in **Marma Chikitsa Practice**

- sīmanta1 (nasamula) = root of the nose at the top, just below sthapani
- sīmanta2 (kapāla) = hairline center in line with sthapani, at top of forehead
- simanta3 (vishnurandhra) = 4 angula anterior from adhipati
- adhipati (brahmarandhra, also known as mūrdhni) = the topmost crown
- sīmanta4 (shivarandhra) = 4 angula posterior from adhipati, the shikha or ponytail area
- sīmanta5 (manyāmula) = the depression at back of head in midline of earlobes

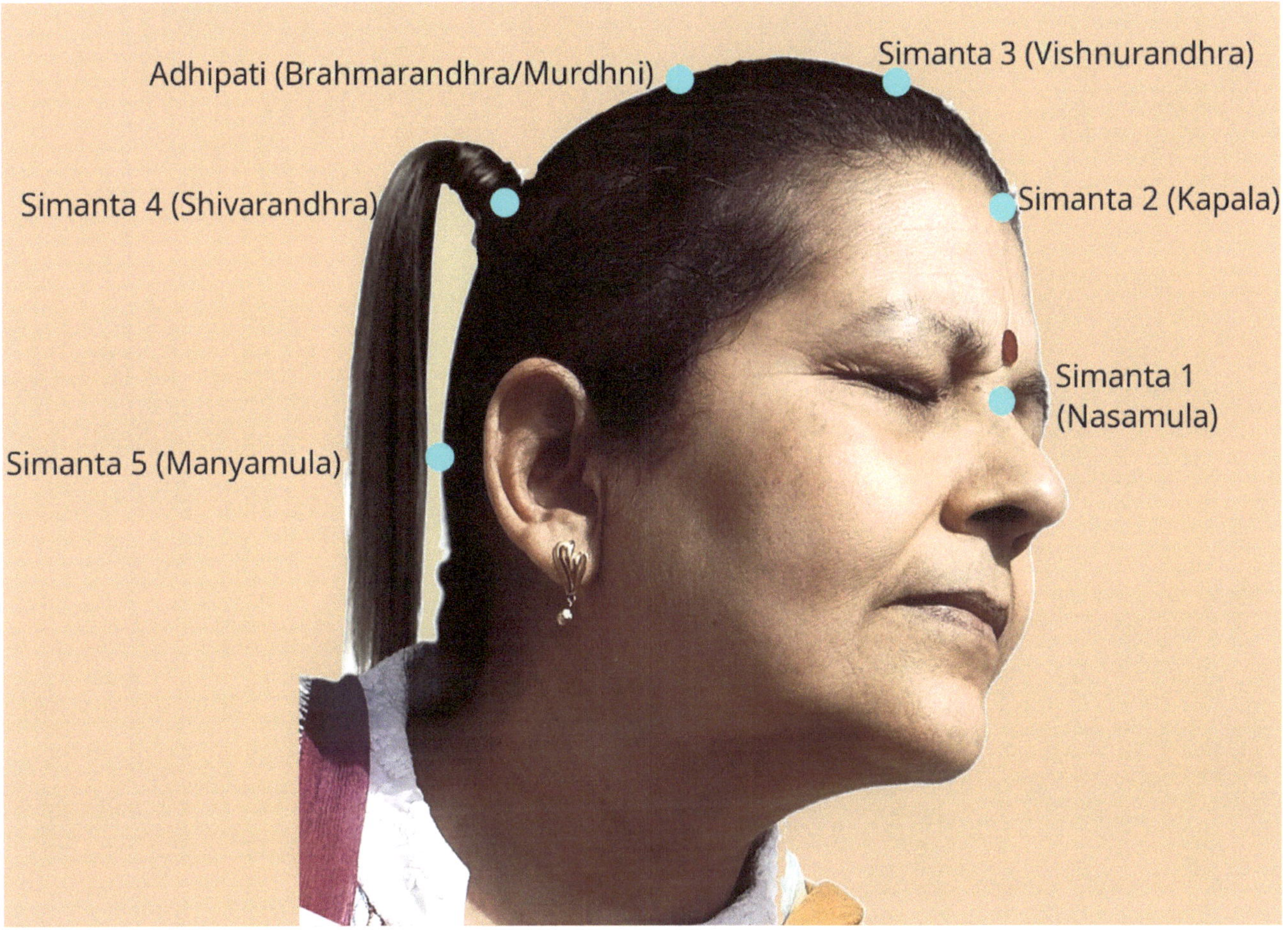

Figure 26 Marma Points on Skull in Practice

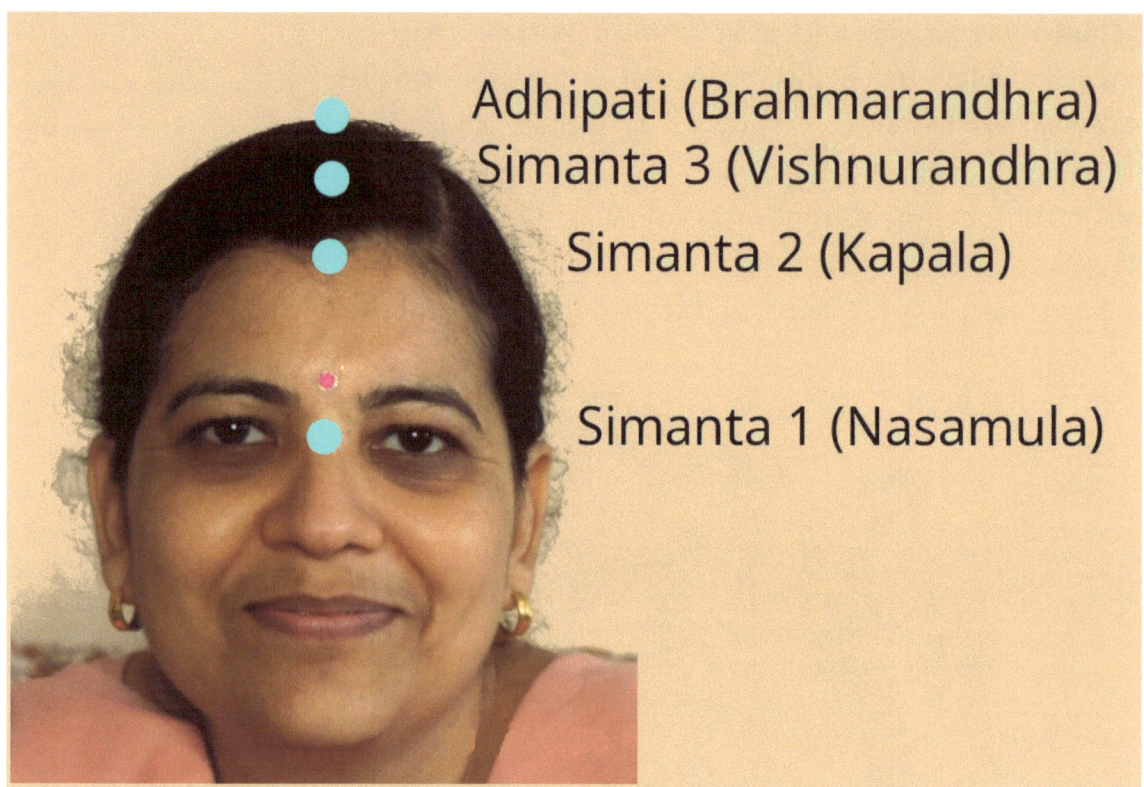

Figure 27 Marma Points Simanta (Front View)
Note: The Points Simanta4 and Simanta5 are not visible here, see Rear View.

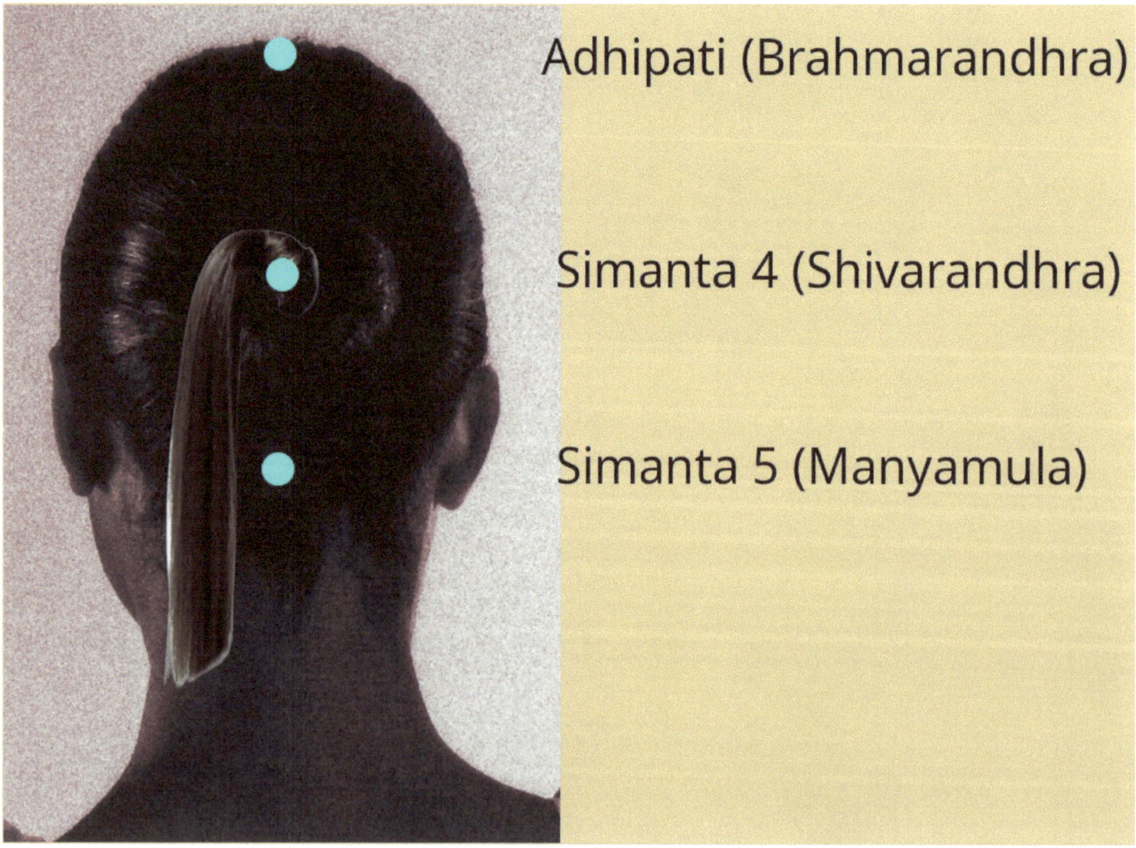

Figure 28 Marma Points Simanta (Rear View)
Note: The Points Simanta 1, 2, 3 are not visible here, see Front View.

Body Tissue type wrt Marma Point Name

तत्र तलहृदयेन्द्रबस्तिगुदस्तनरोहितानि मांसमर्माणि ।

tatra talahṛdayendrabastigudastanarohitāni māṃsamarmāṇi ǀ

Occurrence of marma points in various body tissues.
Marma Point **Names** in type of **Body Tissue मांस māṃsa (Muscle)**:

- तलहृदय talahṛdaya
- इन्द्रबस्ति indrabasti
- गुद guda
- स्तनरोहित stanarohita

Count of 11 Mamsa Marma Points.

नीलधमनीमातृकाश्टृङ्गाटकापाङ्गस्थपनीफणस्तनमूलापलापापस्तम्भहृदयनाभिपार्श्वसन्धिबृहतीलोहिताक्षोर्व्यः सिरामर्माणि ।
nīladhamanīmātṛkāśṛṅgāṭakāpāṅgasthapanīphaṇastanamūlāpalāpāpastambhahṛdayanābhipārśvasandhib ṛhatīlohitākṣorvyaḥ sirāmarmāṇi ǀ

Marma Point **Names** in type of **Body Tissue सिरा sirā (Tube Vein or Artery)**:

- नीला nīlā (pair)
- धमनी dhamanī (pair), (also called manya)
- मातृका mātṛkā (eight)
- शृङ्गाट śṛṅgāṭaka (four)
- अपाङ्ग apāṅga (pair)
- स्थपनी sthapanī
- फण phaṇa (pair)
- स्तनमूल stanamūla (pair)
- अपलाप apalāpa (pair)
- अपस्तम्भ apastambha (pair)
- हृदय hṛdaya
- नाभि nābhi
- पार्श्वसन्धि pārśvasandhi (pair)
- बृहती bṛhatī (pair)
- लोहिताक्ष lohitākṣa (pair + pair)
- ऊर्वी ūrvī (pair + pair)

Count of 41 Sira Marma Points.

आणिविटपकक्षधरकूर्चकूर्चशिरोबस्तिक्षिप्रांसविधुरोत्क्षेपाः स्नायुमर्माणि ।

āṇiviṭapakakṣadharakūrcakūrcaśirobastikṣiprāṃsavidhurotkṣepāḥ snāyumarmāṇi I

Marma Point **Names** in type of **Body Tissue स्नायु snāyu (Nerve/Tendon)**:

- आणि āṇi (pair + pair)
- विटप viṭapa (pair)
- कक्षधर kakṣadhara (pair)
- कूर्च kūrca (pair + pair)
- कूर्चशिर kūrcaśira (pair + pair)
- बस्ति basti
- क्षिप्र kṣiprā (pair + pair)
- अंस aṃsa (pair)
- विधुर vidhura (pair)
- उत्क्षेप utkṣepa (pair)

Count of 27 Snayu Marma Points.

कटीकतरुणनितम्बांसफलकशङ्खास्त्वस्थिमर्माणि ।

kaṭīkataruṇanitambāṃsaphalakaśaṅkhāstvasthimarmāṇi I

Marma Point **Names** in type of **Body Tissue अस्थि asthi (Bone)**:

- कटीकतरुण kaṭīkataruṇa (pair)
- नितम्ब nitamba (pair)
- अंसफलक aṃsaphalaka (pair)
- शङ्ख śaṅkha (pair)

Count of 8 Asthi Marma Points.

जानुकूर्परसीमन्ताधिपतिगुल्फमणिबन्धकुकुन्दरावर्तकृकाटिकाश्चेति सन्धिमर्माणि ॥ ८ ॥

jānukūrparasīmantādhipatigulphamaṇibandhakukundarāvartakṛkāṭikāśceti sandhimarmāṇi II 8 II

Marma Point **Names** in type of **Body Tissue सन्धि sandhi (Joint)**:

- जानु jānu (pair)
- कूर्पर kūrpara (pair)
- सीमन्त sīmanta (five)
- अधिपति adhipati
- गुल्फ gulpha (pair)
- मणिबन्ध maṇibandha (pair)
- कुकुन्दर kukundara (pair)
- आवर्त āvarta (pair)
- कृकाटिका kṛkāṭikā (pair)

Count of 20 Sandhi Marma Points.

Body Injurious Condition wrt Marma Point Name

तान्येतानि पञ्चविकल्पानि भवन्ति । तद्यथा सद्यःप्राणहराणि कालान्तरप्राणहराणि विशल्यघ्नानि वैकल्यकराणि रुजाकराणि चेति ।

tānyetāni pañcavikalpāni bhavanti | tadyathā sadyaḥprāṇaharāṇi kālāntaraprāṇaharāṇi viśalyaghnāni vaikalyakarāṇi rujākarāṇi ceti |

Marma Point injuries give rise to 5 **states** of the Body:

- सद्यःप्राणहराणि sadyaḥprāṇaharāṇi = which proves instantly fatal *(so no help can be given)*
- kālāntaraprāṇaharāṇi = may prove fatal after a while *(proper help should arrive in time)*
- viśalyaghnāni = a foreign body gets lodged at a Marma point and its extraction proves fatal
- वैकल्यकराणि vaikalyakarāṇi = which causes long term disability. i.e., non-fatal
- रुजाकराणि rujākarāṇi = which causes intense pain i.e. non-fatal

तत्र सद्यःप्राणहराण्येकोनविंशतिः कालान्तरप्राणहराणि त्रयस्त्रिंशत् त्रीणि विशल्यघ्नानि चतुश्चत्वारिंशद्वैकल्यकराणि अष्टौ रुजाकराणीति ॥ ९ ॥

tatra sadyaḥprāṇaharāṇyekonaviṃśatiḥ kālāntaraprāṇaharāṇi trayastriṃśat trīṇi viśalyaghnāni catuścatvāriṃśadvaikalyakarāṇi aṣṭau rujākarāṇīti || 9 ||

Marma Point **count** wrt injurious **Body Conditions**:

- sadyaḥprāṇaharāṇi = instantly fatal = 19 Marmas
- kālāntaraprāṇaharāṇi = fatal after a while = 33 Marmas
- viśalyaghnāni = extraction of a foreign body lodged at a Marma point proves fatal = 3 Marmas
- vaikalyakarāṇi = long term disability = 44 Marmas
- rujākarāṇi = intense pain = 8 Marmas

Total Count of 107 Marma Points.

भवन्ति चात्र शृङ्गाटकान्यधिपतिः शङ्खौ कण्ठसिरा गुदम् । हृदयं बस्तिनाभ्यौ च घ्नन्ति सद्यो हतानि तु ॥ १० ॥

bhavanti cātra śṛṅgāṭakānyadhipatiḥ śaṅkhau kaṇṭhasirā gudam | hṛdayaṃ bastinābhyau ca ghnanti sadyo hatāni tu || 10 ||

Marma Point **names** wrt **Body Condition** sadyaḥprāṇahara = instantly fatal:
sadyaḥprāṇaharāṇi = instantly fatal = 19 Marmas

- śṛṅgāṭaka (four)
- adhipati
- śaṅkha (pair)
- kaṇṭhasirā = mātrika (eight)
- guda
- hṛdaya
- basti
- nābhi

वक्षोमर्माणि सीमन्ततलक्षिप्रेन्द्रबस्तयः । कटीकतरुणे सन्धी पार्श्वजौ बृहती च या । नितम्बाविति चैतानि कालान्तरहराणि तु ॥ ११ ॥
vakṣomarmāṇi sīmantatalakṣiprendrabastayaḥ | kaṭīkataruṇe sandhī pārśvajau bṛhatī ca yā | nitambāviti caitāni kālāntaraharāṇi tu || 11 ||

Marma Point **names** wrt **Body Condition** kālāntaraprāṇahara = fatal after a while:
kālāntaraprāṇaharāṇi = fatal after a while = 33 Marmas

- vakṣo-marmāṇi = any Chest and Abdomen Marmas not included in sadyaḥprāṇaharāṇi
  - i.e., stanamūla (pair), stanarohita (pair), apalāpa (pair), apastambha (pair)
- sīmanta (five)
- talahṛdaya (pair + pair)
- kṣipra (pair + pair)
- indrabasti (pair + pair)
- kaṭīkataruṇa (pair)
- pārśvasandhī (pair)
- bṛhatī (pair)
- nitamba (pair)

उत्क्षेपौ स्थपनी चैव विशल्यघ्नानि निर्दिशेत् ॥ १२ ॥

utkṣepau sthapanī caiva viśalyaghnāni nirdiśet || 12 ||

Marma Point **names** wrt **Body Condition** viśalyaghna = fatal upon extraction of foreign matter:
viśalyaghnāni = extraction of foreign body at a Marma point proves fatal = 3 Marmas

- utkṣepa (pair)
- sthapanī

लोहिताक्षाणि जानूर्वीकूर्चविटपकूर्पराः । कुकुन्दरे कक्षधरे विधुरे सकृकाटिके ॥ १३ ॥
अंसांसफलकापाङ्गा नीले मन्ये फणौ तथा । वैकल्यकरणान्याहुरावर्तौ द्वौ तथैव च ॥ १४ ॥

lohitākṣāṇi jānūrvīkūrcaviṭapakūrparāḥ | kukundare kakṣadhare vidhure sakṛkāṭike || 13 ||

aṃsāṃsaphalakāpāṅgā nīle manye phaṇau tathā | vaikalyakaraṇānyāhurāvartau dvau tathaiva ca || 14

Marma Point **names** wrt **Body Condition** vaikalyakara = long term restlessness:
vaikalyakarāṇi = long term disability = 44 Marmas

- lohitākṣa (pair + pair)
- āṇi (pair + pair)
- jānu (pair)
- ūrvī (pair + pair)
- kūrca (pair + pair)
- viṭapa (pair)
- kūrparā (pair)
- kukundara (pair)
- kakṣadhara (pair)
- vidhura (pair)
- kṛkāṭika (pair)

- aṃsa (pair)
- aṃsaphalaka (pair)
- apāṅga (pair)
- nīlā (pair)
- manyā (pair)
- phaṇa (pair)
- āvarta (pair)

गुल्फौ द्वौ मणिबन्धौ द्वौ द्वे द्वे कूर्चशिरांसि च रुजाकराणि ।

gulphau dvau maṇibandhau dvau dve dve kūrcaśirāṃsi ca rujākarāṇi |

Marma Point **names** wrt **Body Condition** rujākara = intense pain:
rujākarāṇi = intense pain = 8 Marmas

- gulpha (pair)
- maṇibandha (pair)
- kūrcaśira (pair + pair)

जानीयादष्टावेतानि बुद्धिमान् । क्षिप्राणि विद्धमात्राणि घ्नन्ति कालान्तरेण च ॥ १५ ॥

jānīyādaṣṭāvetāni buddhimān | kṣiprāṇi viddhamātrāṇi ghnanti kālāntareṇa ca || 15 ||

kṣipra (pair + pair) enumerated earlier, is given here again to emphasize that fatality can be prevented and injurious body condition can be fully healed, if attended to in time properly by the wise.

This goes for the four body conditions viz. kālāntaraprāṇaharāṇi, viśalyaghnāni, vaikalyakarāṇi, rujākarāṇi.

An alternate explanation of this verse is that kṣipra enumerated under kālāntaraprāṇaharāṇi (fatal after some duration) may prove to be sadyaḥprāṇaharāṇi (instantly fatal) at times.

Definition of Marma

मर्माणि मांससिरास्नाय्वस्थिसन्धिसन्निपाताः तेषु स्वभावत एव विशेषेण प्राणास्तिष्ठन्ति । तस्मान्मर्मस्वभिहतास्तांस्तान् भावानापद्यन्ते ॥ १६ ॥

marmāṇi māṃsasirāsnāyvasthisandhisannipātāḥ teṣu svabhāvata eva viśeṣeṇa prāṇāstiṣṭhanti | tasmānmarmasvabhihatāstāṃstān bhāvānāpadyante || 16 ||

Marma is now defined. It is that precise spot in the Body

- where the Prana flow is very high
- where the Consciousness in strongly felt
- which is a Meeting point of the 5 types of body tissues viz. MĀṂSA = Muscles Nerves, SIRĀ = Veins Arteries, SNĀYU = Ligaments Tendons, ASTHI = Bones Teeth Nails Hair, SANDHI = Joints
- where a person feels strong Sensations
- where long term Impressions reside
- which needs to be generally Protected
- which is an entry or exit point for the Soul
- where the soul can be said to be Seated
- where from a person transacts with the Environment and Others
- a point where energy loss or accumulation occurs
- a point from where one may gain or lose
- a point which is sacred or private
- a body part which can cause a big furor in society (if exhibited blatantly)

तत्र सद्यःप्राणहराण्याग्नेयानि, अग्निगुणेष्वाशु क्षीणेषु क्षपयन्ति; कालान्तरप्राणहराणि सौम्याग्नेयानि, अग्निगुणेष्वाशु क्षीणेषु क्रमेण च सोमगुणेषु कालान्तरेण क्षपयन्ति; विशल्यप्राणहराणि वायव्यानि, शल्यमुखावरुद्धो यावदन्तर्वायुस्तिष्ठति तावज्जीवति, उद्धृतमात्रे तु शल्ये मर्मस्थानाश्रितो वायुर्निष्क्रामति, तस्मात् सशल्यो जीवत्युद्धृतशल्यो म्रियते (पाकात्पतितशल्यो वा जीवति); वैकल्यकराणि सौम्यानि, सोमो हि स्थिरत्वाच्छैत्याच्च प्राणावलम्बनं करोति; रुजाकराण्यग्निवायुगुणभूयिष्ठानि, विशेषतश्च तौ रुजाकरौ; पाञ्चभौतिकीं च रुजामाहुरेके ॥ १७ ॥

केचिदाहुर्मांसादीनां पञ्चानामपि समस्तानां विवृद्धानां समवायात् सद्यःप्राणहराणि, एकहीनानामल्पानां वा कालान्तरप्राणहराणि, द्विहीनानां विशल्यप्राणहराणि, त्रिहीनानां वैकल्यकराणि, एकस्मिन्नेव रुजाकराणीति । नैवं, यतोऽस्थिमर्मस्वप्यभिहतेषु शोणितागमनं भवति ॥ १८ ॥

चतुर्विधा यास्तु सिराः शरीरे प्रायेण ता मर्मसु सन्निविष्टाः । स्नाय्वस्थिमांसानि तथैव सन्धीन् सन्तर्प्य देहं प्रतिपालयन्ति ।
ततः क्षते मर्मणि ताः प्रवृद्धः समन्ततो वायुरभिस्तृणोति । विवर्धमानस्तु स मातरिश्वा रुजः सुतीव्राः प्रतनोति काये ॥ १९ ॥
रुजाभिभूतं तु ततः शरीरं प्रलीयते नश्यति चास्य सञ्ज्ञा । अतो हि शल्यं विनिहर्तुमिच्छन्मर्माणि यत्नेन परीक्ष्य कर्षेत् ॥ २० ॥
एतेन शेषं व्याख्यातम् ॥ २१ ॥

तत्र सद्यःप्राणहरमन्ते विद्धं कालान्तरेण मारयति, कालान्तरप्राणहरमन्ते विद्धं वैकल्यमापादयति, विशल्यघ्नं वैकल्यकरं च भवति, वैकल्य करं कालान्तरेण क्लेशयति रुजां च करोति, रुजाकरमतीव्रवेदनं भवति ॥ २२ ॥

तत्र सद्यःप्राणहराणि सप्तरात्राभ्यन्तरान्मारयन्ति, कालान्तरप्राणहराणि पक्षान्मासाद्वा, तेष्वपि तु क्षिप्राणि कदाचिदाशु मारयन्ति, विशल्यप्राणहराणि वैकल्यकराणि च कदाचिदत्यभिहतानि मारयन्ति ॥ २३ ॥

Sushruta's 107 Marma Points anatomically grouped 44+12+14+37

44 Marma Points अत ऊर्ध्वं सक्थिमर्माणि व्याख्यास्यामः

तत्र पादस्याङ्गुष्ठाङ्गुल्योर्मध्ये क्षिप्रं[2] नाम मर्म, तत्र विद्धस्याक्षेपकेण मरणं; मध्यमाङ्गुलीमनुपूर्वेण मध्ये पादतलस्य तलहृदयं[2] नाम , तत्र रुजाभिर्मरणं; क्षिप्रस्योपरिष्टादुभयतः कूर्चो[2] नाम, तत्र पादस्य भ्रमणवेपने भवतः; गुल्फसन्धेरध उभयतः कूर्चशिरः[2], तत्र रुजाशोफौ; पादजङ्घयोः सन्धाने गुल्फः[2], तत्र रुजः स्तब्धपादता खञ्जता वा; पार्ष्णिं प्रति जङ्घामध्ये इन्द्रबस्तिः[2], तत्र शोणितक्षयेण मरणं; जङ्घोर्वोः सन्धाने जानु[2], तत्र खञ्जता; जानुन ऊर्ध्वमुभयतस्त्र्यङ्गुलमाणी[2], तत्र शोफाभिवृद्धिः स्तब्धसक्थिता च; ऊरुमध्ये ऊर्वी[2], तत्र शोणितक्षयात् सक्थिशोषः ; ऊर्व्या ऊर्ध्वमधो वङ्क्षणसन्धेरूरुमूले लोहिताक्षं[2], तत्र लोहितक्षयेण मरणं पक्षाघातो वा; वङ्क्षणवृषणयोरन्तरे विटपं[2], तत्र षाण्ढ्यमल्पशुक्रता वा भवति; एवमेतान्येकादश eleven सक्थिमर्माणि व्याख्यातानि । एतेनेतरसक्थि बाहू च व्याख्यातौ । विशेषतस्तु यानि सक्थि गुल्फ-जानु-विटपानि, तानि बाहौ मणिबन्ध[2]-कूर्पर[2]-कक्षधराणि[2] ; यथा वङ्क्षणवृषणयोरन्तरे विटपमेवं वक्षःकक्षयोर्मध्ये कक्षधरं, तस्मिन् विद्धे त एवोपद्रवाः; विशेषतस्तु मणिबन्धे कुण्ठता, कूर्पराख्ये कुणिः, कक्षधरे पक्षाघातः । एवमेतानि चतुश्चत्वारिंश forty four च्छाखासु मर्माणि व्याख्यातानि ॥ २४ ॥ (*Note: ऊर्वी also spelt उर्वी*)

Book.Chapter.Verse = Sharira Sthana.Marmani.Verse = 4.6.Verse = 4.6.24

Now is described the Marma Points in the **Leg and Foot.** Verse No 4.6.24				No of Points in
Marma No	**Marma Location and Point**	**Marma Name**	**SNo**	**each leg**
1, 2	पादस्याङ्गुष्ठाङ्गुल्योर्मध्ये क्षिप्रं = क्षिप्र junction of big toe & next toe finger	kṣipra (kshipra)	1	1
3, 4	मध्यमाङ्गुलीमनुपूर्वेण मध्ये पादतलस्य तलहृदयं = तलहृदय center of sole of foot	talahṛdaya (talahridaya)	2	1
5, 6	क्षिप्रस्योपरिष्टादुभयतः कूर्चो = कूर्च extremity of big toe on the foot, two angula posterior from kṣipra	kūrca (kurcha)	3	1
7, 8	गुल्फसन्धेरध उभयतः कूर्चशिरः = कूर्चशिर junction center of foot with leg	kūrcaśira (kurchashira)	4	1
9, 10	पादजङ्घयोः सन्धाने गुल्फः = गुल्फ below the ankle bone	gulpha	5	1
11, 12	पार्ष्णिं प्रति जङ्घामध्ये इन्द्रबस्तिः = इन्द्रबस्ति in the calf center, 12 angula posterior from ankle bone	indrabasti	6	1
13, 14	जङ्घोर्वोः सन्धाने जानुः = जानु at junction of knee joint with calf	jānu (janu)	7	1
15, 16	जानुन ऊर्ध्वमुभयतस्त्र्यङ्गुलम् आणी = आणि 3 angula above knee joint	āṇi (ani)	8	1
17, 18	ऊरुमध्ये ऊर्वी = ऊर्वी at center of thigh	ūrvī (urvi)	9	1
19, 20	उर्व्या ऊर्ध्वमधो वङ्क्षणसन्धेरूरुमूले लोहिताक्षं = लोहिताक्ष in the groin junction at root of thigh	lohitākṣa (lohitaksha)	10	1

21, 22	वङ्क्षणवृषणयोरन्तरे विटपं = विटप between the inguinal canal and scrotum	viṭapa (vitapa)	11	1
			Sum	**11**
4.6.24 विशेषतस्तु यानि सक्थ्नि गुल्फ-जानु-विटपानि, तानि बाहौ मणिबन्ध-कूर्पर-कक्षधराणि । The points in Leg named गुल्फ-जानु-विटप are mirrored as मणिबन्ध-कूर्पर-कक्षधर in the Arm.				
These **eleven** points in one leg are mirrored in the other leg also. Hence a total of 11x2 = **22 Marmas**.				

Now is described the Marma Points in the **Arm and Hand.** Verse No 4.6.24				No of Points
Marma No	**Marma Location and Point**	**Marma Name**	**SNo**	**in each arm**
23, 24	पादस्याङ्गुष्ठाङ्गुल्योर्मध्ये क्षिप्रं = क्षिप्र junction of thumb & index finger	kṣipra (kshipra)	1	1
25, 26	मध्यमाङ्गुलीमनुपूर्वेण मध्ये पादतलस्य तलहृदयं = तलहृदय center of palm	talahṛdaya (talahridaya)	2	1
27, 28	क्षिप्रस्योपरिष्टादुभयतः कूर्चो = कूर्च extremity of thumb on hand, two angula posterior from kṣipra	kūrca (kurcha)	3	1
29, 30	गुल्फसन्धेरध उभयतः कूर्चशिरः = कूर्चशिर junction center of hand with arm	kūrcaśira (kurchashira)	4	1
31, 32	पादजङ्घयोः सन्धाने मणिबन्धः = मणिबन्ध anterior to wrist bone	maṇibandha (manibandha)	5	1
33, 34	पार्ष्णिं प्रति जङ्घामध्ये इन्द्रबस्तिः = इन्द्रबस्ति in forearm center, 12 angula posterior from wrist bone	indrabasti	6	1
35, 36	जङ्घोर्वोः सन्धाने कूर्परः = कूर्पर at junction of elbow joint with forearm	kūrpara (kurpara)	7	1
37, 38	जानुन ऊर्ध्वमुभयतस्त्र्यङ्गुलम् आणी = आणि 3 angula above elbow joint	āṇi (ani)	8	1
39, 40	ऊरुमध्ये ऊर्वी = ऊर्वी midpoint of upper arm	ūrvī (urvi)	9	1
41, 42	उर्व्या ऊर्ध्वमधो वङ्क्षणसन्धेरूरुमूले लोहिताक्षं = लोहिताक्ष the armpit junction at root of arm	lohitākṣa (lohitaksha)	10	1
43, 44	वङ्क्षणवृषणयोरन्तरे कक्षधरं = कक्षधर above the armpit junction with torso	kakṣadhara (kakshadhara)	11	1
			Sum	**11**
4.6.24 विशेषतस्तु यानि सक्थ्नि गुल्फ-जानु-विटपानि, तानि बाहौ मणिबन्ध-कूर्पर-कक्षधराणि । The points in Leg named गुल्फ-जानु-विटप are mirrored as मणिबन्ध-कूर्पर-कक्षधरा in the Arm.				
These **eleven** points seen in one leg are mirrored in the other leg also. As well as in both arms. Hence a total of 11x2x2 = **44 Marmas**.				

12 Marma Points अत ऊर्ध्वमुदरोरसोर्मर्माण्यनुव्याख्यास्यामः

तत्र वातवर्चोनिरसनं स्थूलान्त्रप्रतिबद्धं गुदं[1] नाम मर्म, तत्र सद्योमरणं; अल्पमांसशोणितोऽभ्यन्तरतः कट्यां मूत्राशयो बस्तिः[1], तत्रापि सद्योमरणमश्मरीव्रणादृते, तत्राप्युभयतो भिन्ने न जीवति , एकतो भिन्ने मूत्रस्रावी व्रणो भवति, स तु यत्नेनोपक्रान्तो रोहति; पक्वामाशययोर्मध्ये सिराप्रभवा नाभिः[1], तत्रापि सद्यो मरणं; स्तनयोर्मध्यमधिष्ठायोरस्यामाशयद्वारं सत्त्वरजस्तमसामधिष्ठानं हृदयं[1], तत्रापि सद्य एव मरणं; स्तनयोरधस्ताद् द्व्यङ्गुलमुभयतः स्तनमूले[2], तत्र कफपूर्णकोष्ठतया (कासश्वासाभ्यां) म्रियते; स्तनचूचुकयोरूर्ध्वं द्व्यङ्गुलमुभयतः स्तनरोहितौ[2], तत्र लोहितपूर्णकोष्ठतया कासश्वासाभ्यां च म्रियते; अंसकूटयोरधस्तात् पार्श्वोपरिभागयोरपलापौ[2] नाम, तत्र रक्तेन पूयभावं गतेन मरणं; उभयत्रोरसो नाड्यौ वातवहे अपस्तम्भौ[2] नाम, तत्र वातपूर्णकोष्ठतया कासश्वासाभ्यां च मरणम् ;

एवमेतान्युदरोरसोर्द्वादश twelve stomach मर्माणि व्याख्यातानि ॥ २५ ॥

Now is described the Marma Points in the **Chest and Abdomen.** Verse No 4.6.25				
Marma No	**Marma Location Point**	**Marma Name**	**SNo**	**No of Points**
45	वातवर्चोनिरसनं स्थूलान्त्रप्रतिबद्धं गुदं = गुद at anus	guda	1	1
46	अल्पमांसशोणितोऽभ्यन्तरतः कट्यां मूत्राशयो बस्तिः = बस्ति at bladder	basti	2	1
47	पक्वामाशययोर्मध्ये सिराप्रभवा नाभिः = नाभि at navel	nābhi (nabhi)	3	1
48	स्तनयोर्मध्यमधिष्ठायोरस्यामाशयद्वारं सत्त्वरजस्तमसामधिष्ठानं हृदयं = हृदय at heart center (chest midline between the breasts)	hṛdaya (hridaya)	4	1
49, 50	स्तनयोः अधस्ताद् द्व्यङ्गुलमुभयतः स्तनमूले = स्तनमूल 2 angula below nipple	stanamūla (stanamula)	5	2
51, 52	स्तन-चूचुकयोः ऊर्ध्वं द्व्यङ्गुलमुभयतः स्तनरोहितौ = स्तनरोहित 2 angula above nipple	stanarohita	6	2
53, 54	अंसकूटयोः अधस्तात् पार्श्वोपरिभागयोर् अपलापौ = अपलाप at upper ribcage below shoulder ball	apalāpa (apalapa)	7	2
55, 56	उभयत्र उरसो नाड्यौ वातवहे अपस्तम्भौ = अपस्तम्भ on bronchial tubes of upper chest area	apastambha	8	2
			Sum	**12**
Thus **12 Marma** points in **Chest and Abdomen**				

14 Marma Points अत ऊर्ध्वं पृष्ठमर्माणि व्याख्यास्यामः

तत्र पृष्ठवंशमुभयतः प्रतिश्रोणिकाण्डमस्थिनी कटीकतरुणे[2], तत्र शोणितक्षयात् पाण्डुर्विवर्णो हीनरूपश्च म्रियते; पार्श्वयोर्जघनबहिर्भागे पृष्ठवंशमुभयतो कुकुन्दरे[2], तत्र स्पर्शाज्ञानमधःकाये चेष्टोपघातश्च; श्रोणीकाण्डयोरुपर्याशयाच्छादनौ पार्श्वान्तरप्रतिबद्धौ नितम्बौ[2], तत्राधःकायशोषो दौर्बल्याच्च मरणं; अधःपार्श्वान्तरप्रतिबद्धौ जघनपार्श्वमध्ययोस्तिर्यगूर्ध्वं च जघनात् पार्श्वसन्धी[2], तत्र लोहितपूर्णकोष्ठतया म्रियते; स्तनमूलादृजूभयतः पृष्ठवंशस्य बृहती[2], तत्र शोणितातिप्रवृत्तिनिमित्तैरुपद्रवैर्म्रियते; पृष्ठोपरि पृष्ठवंशमुभयतस्त्रिकसम्बद्धे अंसफलके[2], तत्र बाह्वोः[2] स्वापशोषौ ; बाहुमूर्धग्रीवामध्येंऽसपीठस्कन्धबन्धनावंसौ[2], तत्र स्तब्धबाहुता; एवमेतानि चतुर्दश fourteen पृष्ठमर्माणि back व्याख्यातानि ॥ २६ ॥

Now is described the Marma Points in the **Back.** Verse No 4.6.26				
Marma No	**Marma Location Point**	**Marma Name**	**SNo**	**No of Points**
57, 58	पृष्ठवंशमुभयतः प्रतिश्रोणिकाण्डमस्थिनी कटीकतरुणे = कटीकतरुण	kaṭīkataruṇa (katikataruna)	1	2
59, 60	पार्श्वयोर्जघनबहिर्भागे पृष्ठवंशमुभयतो कुकुन्दरे = कुकुन्दर	kukundara	2	2
61, 62	श्रोणीकाण्डयोरुपर्याशयाच्छादनौ पार्श्वान्तरप्रतिबद्धौ नितम्बौ = नितम्ब	nitamba	3	2
63, 64	अधःपार्श्वान्तरप्रतिबद्धौ जघनपार्श्वमध्ययोस्तिर्यगूर्ध्वं च जघनात् पार्श्वसन्धी = पार्श्वसन्धि	pārśvasandhi (parshvasandhi)	4	2
65, 66	स्तनमूलादृजूभयतः पृष्ठवंशस्य बृहती = बृहती	bṛhatī (brihati)	5	2
67, 68	पृष्ठोपरि पृष्ठवंशमुभयतस्त्रिकसम्बद्धे अंसफलके = अंसफलक	aṃsaphalaka (amsaphalaka)	6	2
69, 70	बाहुमूर्धग्रीवामध्येंऽसपीठस्कन्धबन्धनौ अंसौ = अंस	aṃsa (amsa)	7	2
			Sum	**14**
Thus **14 Marma** points in **Back**				

37 Marma Points अत ऊर्ध्वमूर्ध्वजत्रुगतानि व्याख्यास्यामः-

तत्र कण्ठनाडीमुभयतश्चतस्रो four धमन्यो द्वे नीले[2] Nila द्वे च मन्ये[2] Manya व्यत्यासेन , तत्र मूकता स्वरवैकृतमरसग्राहिता च; ग्रीवायामुभयतश्चतस्रः four pairs सिरा मातृकाः[8] SiraMatrika तत्र सद्योमरणं; शिरोग्रीवयोः सन्धाने कृकाटिके[2] Krikatika, तत्र चलमूर्धता; कर्णपृष्ठतोऽधःसंश्रिते विधुरे[2] Vidhura , तत्र बाधिर्यं; घ्राणमार्गमुभयतः स्रोतोमार्गप्रतिबद्धे अभ्यन्तरतः फणे[2] Phana , तत्र गन्धाज्ञानं; भ्रूपुच्छान्तयोरधोऽक्ष्णोर्बाह्यतोऽपाङ्गौ[2] Apanga , तत्रान्ध्यं दृष्ट्युपघातो वा; भ्रुवोरुपरि निम्नयोरावर्तौ[2] Avarta नाम , तत्राप्यान्ध्यं दृष्ट्युपघातो वा; भ्रुवोरन्तयोरुपरि [४८] कर्णललाटयोर्मध्ये शङ्खौ[2] Shankha Temple तत्र सद्योमरणं; शङ्खयोरुपरि केशान्त उत्क्षेपौ[2] Utkshepa तत्र सशल्यो जीवेत् पाकात् पतितशल्यो वा नोद्धृतशल्यः; भ्रुवोर्मध्ये स्थपनी[1] Sthapani तत्रोत्क्षेपवत् ; पञ्च five सन्धयः शिरसि विभक्ताः सीमन्ता[5] Simanta नाम a) Manyamula, b) Shivarandhra c) Vishnurandhra d) Kapala e) , तत्रोन्मादभयचित्तनाशैर्मरणं; घ्राणश्रोत्राक्षिजिह्वासन्तर्पणीनां सिराणां मध्ये सिरासन्निपातः शृङ्गाटकानि[4] Shringataka , तानि चत्वारि four मर्माणि, तत्रापि सद्योमरणं; मस्तकाभ्यन्तरोपरिष्टात् सिरासन्धिसन्निपातो रोमावर्तोऽधिपतिः[1] Adhipati , तत्रापि सद्य एव । एवमेतानि thirty-seven marmas सप्तत्रिंशदूर्ध्वजत्रुगतानि मर्माणि व्याख्यातानि ॥ २७ ॥

Now is described the Marma Points in the **Head and Neck.** Verse No 4.6.27				
M No	Marma Location Point	Marma Name	SNo	No of Points
71-74	कण्ठनाडीमुभयतश्चतस्रो धमन्यो द्वे नीले च मन्ये = 71-72 नीला, 73-74 मन्या	nīlā, manyā (nila, manya)	1, 2	2 pairs = 4
75-82	ग्रीवायामुभयतश्चतस्रः सिरा मातृकाः = मातृका 75-76 = मातृका 1a, b = अक्षक akshaka 77 = मातृका 2a = कण्ठनाडी kaṇṭhanāḍī 78 = मातृका 2b = कण्ठ kaṇṭha 79-80=मातृका 3a, b= पृष्ठग्रीव pṛṣṭhagrīva 81 = मातृका 4a = मन्यामणि manyāmaṇi 82 = मातृका 4b = ग्रीवा grīvā	mātṛkā (matrika) = matrika1a,b = akshaka pair, matrika2a=kanthanadi, matrika2b = kantha, matrika3a,b = prishtagriva pair, matrika4a=manyamani matrika4b = griva	3	4 pairs = 8
83, 84	शिरोग्रीवयोः सन्धाने कृकाटिके = कृकाटिका	kṛkāṭikā (krikatika)	4	1 pair = 2
85, 86	कर्णपृष्ठतोऽधःसंश्रिते विधुरे = विधुर	vidhura	5	1 pair = 2
87, 88	घ्राणमार्गमुभयतः स्रोतोमार्गप्रतिबद्धे अभ्यन्तरतः फणे = फण	phaṇa (phana)	6	1 pair = 2
89, 90	भ्रूपुच्छान्तयोरधोऽक्ष्णोर्बाह्यतः अपाङ्गौ = अपाङ्ग	apāṅga (apanga)	7	1 pair = 2
91, 92	भ्रुवोरुपरि निम्नयोर् आवर्तौ = आवर्त	āvarta (avarta)	8	1 pair = 2
93, 94	भ्रुवोरन्तयोरुपरि कर्णललाटयोर्मध्ये शङ्खौ = शङ्ख	śaṅkha (shankha)	9	1 pair = 2
95, 96	शङ्खयोरुपरि केशान्तः उत्क्षेपौ = उत्क्षेप	utkṣepa (utkshepa)	10	1 pair = 2
97	भ्रुवोर्मध्ये स्थपनी = स्थपनी	sthapanī (sthapani)	11	1
98-101	घ्राण-श्रोत्र-अक्षि-जिह्वा-सन्तर्पणीनां सिराणां मध्ये सिरासन्निपातः शृङ्गाटकानि = शृङ्गाटक 98 = शृङ्गाटक 1a = ओष्ठ, 1b = हनु 99 = शृङ्गाटक 2a,b = कपोलनासा 100= शृङ्गाटक 3a,b = कर्णपालि 101 = शृङ्गाटक 4a,b = कनीनक	śṛṅgāṭaka (shringataka) shringataka1 = oshtha, hanu shringataka2 = kapolanasa pair shringataka3 = karnapali pair shringataka4 = kaninaka pair	13	4
102-106	पञ्च सन्धयः शिरसि विभक्ताः सीमन्ताः =सीमन्त 102 = simanta 1 = नासामूल nāsāmūla 103 = simanta 2 = कपाल kapāla 104 =simanta3=विष्णुरन्ध्र viṣṇurandhra 105 = simanta 4 = शिवरन्ध्र śivarandhra 106 = simanta 5 = मन्यामूल manyāmūla	sīmanta (simanta) simanta1 = nasamula simanta2 = kapala simanta3=vishnurandhra simanta4=shivarandhra simanta5 = manyamula	12	5
107	मस्तकाभ्यन्तरोपरिष्ठात् सिरासन्धिसन्निपातो रोमावर्तः अधिपतिः = अधिपति (ब्रह्मरंध्र / मूर्धनि)	adhipati (brahmarandhra or mūrdhni or crown)	14	1
			Sum	**37**
Thus **37 Marma** points in **Head and Neck**				

Dhamani Matrika Shringataka Simanta Marma Points

Some **Marma** points in **Head and Neck** are **named** and clarified for the Practitioner, as these are not explicitly specified in the Samhita. The SNo are arbitrary for clarity.

dhamanī 2 pairs (धमनी *arteries at neck front*)

71-72 = dhamani 2a, 2b = मन्या **manyā** pair (also called **mantha**)

73-74 = dhamani 1a, 1b = नीला **nīlā** pair (also called **sirāmantha**)

mātṛkā 8 points (4 pairs also called सिरा मातृका **sirā mātṛkā** *nourishing veins in neck*)

75-76 = matrika 1a, 1b (at neck front)= अक्षक **akṣaka** pair

77 = matrika 2a (at neck front)= कण्ठनाडी **kaṇṭhanāḍī**

78 = matrika 2b = कण्ठ **kaṇṭha**

79-80 = matrika 3a, 3b (at neck rear)= पृष्ठग्रीव **pṛṣṭhagrīva** pair

81 = matrika 4a (neck rear)= neck bone मन्यामणि **manyāmaṇi**

82 = matrika 4b = neck ग्रीवा **grīvā**

śṛṅgāṭaka 4 nerves (श्रृङ्गाटक for घ्राण smell, श्रोत्र hearing, अक्षि sight, जिह्वा taste); in practice we use 4 pairs

98 = shringataka 1a, 1b - Related to Tongue – upper lip ओष्ठ **oṣṭha** one, chin हनु **hanu** one

99 = shringataka 2a, 2b - Related to Nose - nostrils कपोल नासा **kapola nāsā** pair

100 = shringataka 3a, 3b - Related to Ears - earlobes कर्णपालि **karṇapāli** pair

101 = shringataka 4a, 4b - Related to Eyes - pupils कनीनका **kanīnakā** pair

Some practitioners use additional points in the face. E.g., Nasaputa, Kapola Madhya, etc.

sīmanta 5 nos (सीमन्त *partitions on skull*), in practice we use the points

102 = simanta 1 = root of nose नासामूल **nāsāmūla**

103 = simanta 2 = top of forehead कपाल **kapāla**

104 = simanta 3 = anterior fontanelle विष्णुरन्ध्र / विष्णुरंध्र **viṣṇurandhra**

105 = simanta 4 = posterior fontanelle शिवरन्ध्र / शिवरंध्र **śivarandhra**

106 = simanta 5 = root of skull मन्यामूल **manyāmūla**

Dimensions of each of Sushruta's 107 Marma Points

<u>भवन्ति चात्र श्लोकाः And these verses</u>

ऊर्व्यः शिरांसि विटपे च सकक्षपार्श्वे एकैकमङ्गुलमितं स्तनपूर्वमूलम् ।

विद्ध्यङ्गुलद्वयमितं मणिबन्धगुल्फं त्रीण्येव जानु सपरं सह कूर्पराभ्याम् ॥ २८ ॥

हृद्बस्तिकूर्चगुदनाभि वदन्ति मूर्ध्नि चत्वारि पञ्च च गले दश यानि च द्वे ।

तानि स्वपाणितलकुञ्चितसम्मितानि शेषाण्यवेहि परिविस्तरतोऽङ्गुलार्धम् ॥ २९ ॥

ūrvyaḥ śirāṃsi viṭape ca sakakṣapārśve ekaikamaṅgulamitaṃ stanapūrvamūlam I

viddhyaṅguladvayamitaṃ maṇibandhagulphaṃ trīṇyeva jānu saparaṃ saha kūrparābhyām II 28 II

hṛdbastikūrcagudanābhi vadanti mūrdhni catvāri pañca ca gale daśa yāni ca dve I

tāni svapāṇitalakuñcitasammitāni śeṣāṇyavehi parivistarato'ṅgulārdham II 29 II

Sushruta now gives the size of each Marma Point, in terms of Finger and Palm measurement. He explicitly mentions the term स्व, i.e., the finger and palm measurements pertain to each specific person. Since people's bodies vary in form, size, appearance, the Marma Practitioner must get an idea of the Client's finger and palm before beginning the therapy. The term मूर्ध्नि used here is interpreted as श्रृङ्गाटक since attached to 4 points. (The term Murdhni is also used to mean Adhipati).

<u>For correct interpretation, we refer to the relevant verses from Ashtanga Hridayam.</u>

तेषां विटपकक्षाधृगुर्व्यः कूर्चशिरांसि च । द्वादश अङ्गुलमानानि Of these, 12 points are of 1 Angula each

द्व्यङ्गुले मणिबन्धने ॥ ६० ॥ गुल्फौ च स्तनमूले च 2 Angula each are Manibandha Gulpha Stanamula

त्र्यङ्गुलं जानुकूर्परम् । 3 Angula each are Janu Kurpara

अपानबस्तिहृन्नाभिनीलाः सीमन्तमातृकाः ॥ ६१ ॥ कूर्चश्रृङ्गाटमन्याश्च त्रिंशदेकेन वर्जिताः । आत्मपाणितलोन्मानाः These points are 1 less than 30, i.e., 29 in number, and size of one's own palm.

शेषाण्यर्द्धाङ्गुलं वदेत् ॥ ६२ ॥ पञ्चाशत्षट् च मर्माणि, तिलव्रीहिसमान्यपि । Rest are ½ Angula each, 56 in number. We can also say these rest are the size of a grain of rice each.

Verse	Marma	Dimension	Marma Point	Size	Points
4.6.28	ऊर्व्यः शिरांसि विटपे च सकक्षपार्श्वे एकैकमङ्गुलमितं	एक-एकम्-अङ्गुलम् इतं	ऊर्वी$^{2+2}$ urvi, कूर्चशिर$^{2+2}$ kurchashira, विटप^{2} vitapa, कक्षधर^{2} kakshadhara	1 angula each	2+2+2+2+2 +2 = 12
4.6.28	स्तनपूर्वमूलम् विद्ध्यङ्गुलद्वयमितं मणिबन्धगुल्फं	विद्धि-अङ्गुल-द्वयम् इतं	स्तनमूल stanamula, मणिबन्ध manibandha, गुल्फ gulpha	2 angula each	3x2 = 6
4.6.28	त्रीण्येव जानु सपरं सह कूर्पराभ्याम्	त्रीणि एव	जानु janu, कूर्पर kurpara	3 angula each	2x2 = 4
4.6.29	हृद्बस्तिकूर्चगुदनाभि वदन्ति मूर्ध्नि चत्वारि पञ्च च गले दश यानि च द्वे । hridaya, basti, kurcha, guda, nabhi	तानि स्व-पाणितल-कुञ्चितसम्मितानि shringataka, simanta	हृदय, बस्ति, leg कूर्च^{2}, arm कूर्च^{2} , गुद , नाभि, श्रृङ्गाटक^{4}, सीमन्त^{5}, matrika & nila neck^{10} , dhamani manya^{2}	Palm size each (of Self)	1+1+2+2+1 +1+4+5+10 +2 = 29
4.6.29	शेषाण्यवेहि	परिविस्तरतः अङ्गुल-अर्धम्	all remaining	½ angula each	56
				total	**107**

Angula measurement is derived from अङ्गुलि Aṅguli = Finger. One Angula is precisely the horizontal width of the **middle segment of middle finger** of a person. This measurement is **relative** to the body of the person, i.e., 1 angula will vary in exact size from person to person, since width of each person's finger will vary. Similarly **palm** of each person.

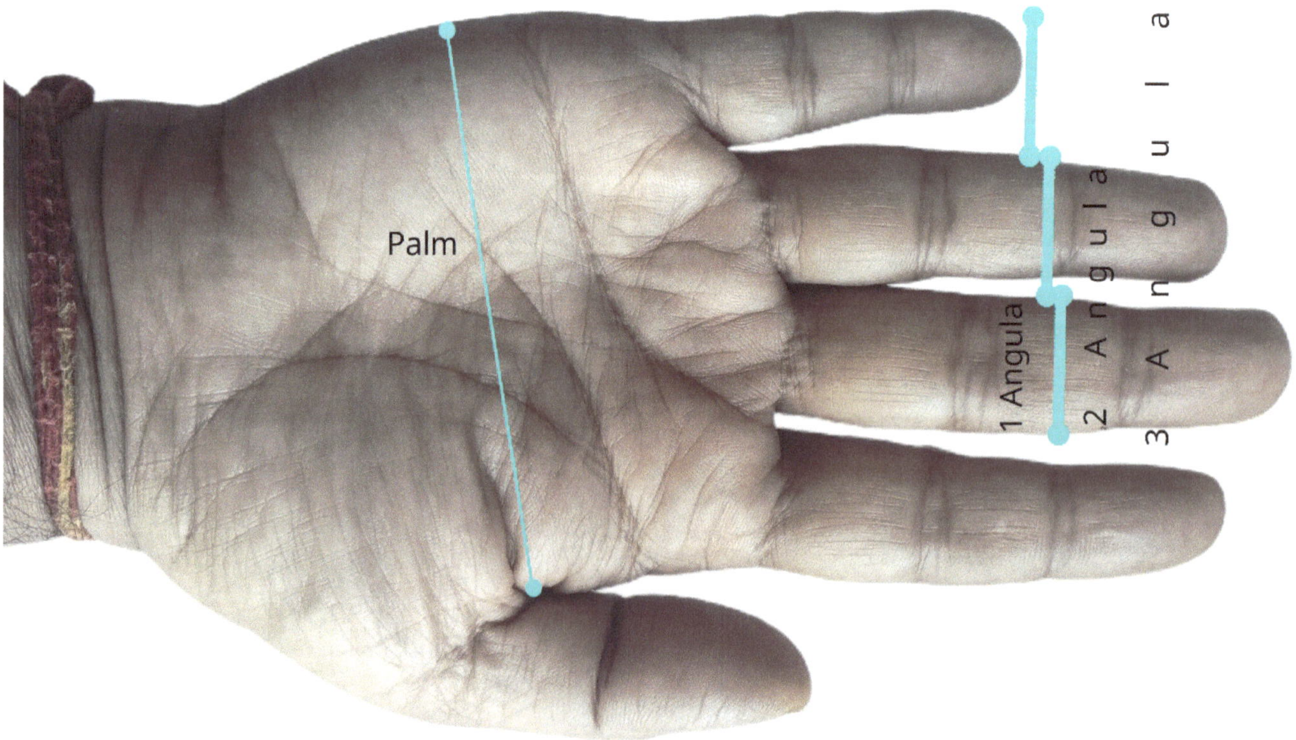

एतत्प्रमाणमभिवीक्ष्य वदन्ति तज्ज्ञाः शस्त्रेण कर्मकरणं परिहृत्य कार्यम् ।
पार्श्वाभिघातितमपीह निहन्ति मर्म तस्माद्धि मर्मसदनं परिवर्जनीयम् ॥ ३० ॥
छिन्नेषु पाणिचरणेषु सिरा नराणां सङ्कोचमीयुरसृगल्पमतो निरेति ।
प्राप्यामितव्यसनमुग्रमतो मनुष्याः सञ्च्छिन्नशाखतरुवन्निधनं न यान्ति ॥ ३१ ॥
क्षिप्रेषु तत्र सतलेषु हतेषु रक्तं गच्छत्यतीव पवनश्च रुजं करोति ।
एवं विनाशमुपयान्ति हि तत्र विद्धा वृक्षा इवायुधनिपातनिकृत्तमूलाः ॥ ३२ ॥
तस्मात् तयोरभिहतस्य तु पाणिपादं छेत्तव्यमाशु मणिबन्धनगुल्फदेशे ।
मर्माणि शल्यविषयार्धमुदाहरन्ति यस्माच्च मर्मसु हता न भवन्ति सद्यः ।
जीवन्ति तत्र यदि वैद्यगुणेन केचित् ते प्राप्नुवन्ति विकलत्वमसंशयं हि ॥ ३३ ॥
सम्भिन्नजर्जरितकोष्ठशिरःकपाला जीवन्ति शस्त्रनिहतैश्च शरीरदेशैः ।
छिन्नैश्च सक्थिभुजपादकरैरशेषैर्येषां न मर्मसु कृता विविधाः प्रहाराः ॥ ३४ ॥
सोममारुततेजांसि रजःसत्त्वतमांसि च । मर्मसु प्रायशः पुंसां भूतात्मा चावतिष्ठते ॥ ३५ ॥
मर्मस्वभिहतास्तस्मान्न जीवन्ति शरीरिणः । इन्द्रियार्थेष्वसम्प्राप्तिर्मनोबुद्धिविपर्ययः ॥ ३६ ॥
रुजश्च विविधास्तीव्रा भवन्त्याशुहरे हते । हते कालान्तरघ्ने तु ध्रुवं धातुक्षयो नृणाम् ॥ ३७ ॥
ततो धातुक्षयाज्जन्तुर्वेदनाभिश्च नश्यति । हते वैकल्यजनने केवलं वैद्यनैपुणात् ॥ ३८ ॥
शरीरं क्रियया युक्तं विकलत्वमवाप्नुयात् । विशल्यघ्ने तु विज्ञेयं पूर्वोक्तं यच्च कारणम् । ३९
रुजाकराणि मर्माणि क्षतानि विविधा रुजः । कुर्वन्त्यन्ते च वैकल्यं कुवैद्यवशगो यदि ॥ ४० ॥
छेदभेदाभिघातेभ्यो दहनाद्दारणादपि । उपघातं विजानीयान्मर्मणां तुल्यलक्षणम् ॥ ४१ ॥
मर्माभिघातस्तु न कश्चिदस्ति योऽल्पात्ययो वाऽपि निरत्ययो वा । प्रायेण मर्मस्वभिताडितास्तु वैकल्यमृच्छन्त्यथवा म्रियन्ते ॥ ४२ ॥
मर्माण्यधिष्ठाय हि ये विकारा मूर्च्छन्ति काये विविधा नराणाम् । प्रायेण ते कृच्छ्रतमा भवन्ति नरस्य यत्नैरपि साध्यमानाः ॥ ४३ ॥

॥ इति सुश्रुतसंहितायां शारीरस्थाने प्रत्येकमर्मनिर्देशशारीरं नाम षष्ठोऽध्यायः ॥

END of the 6th **Chapter** named **Marma Directive** of the **Sharira Sthana Section** of Sushruta Samhita.

Sushruta's 107 Marma Points Collated

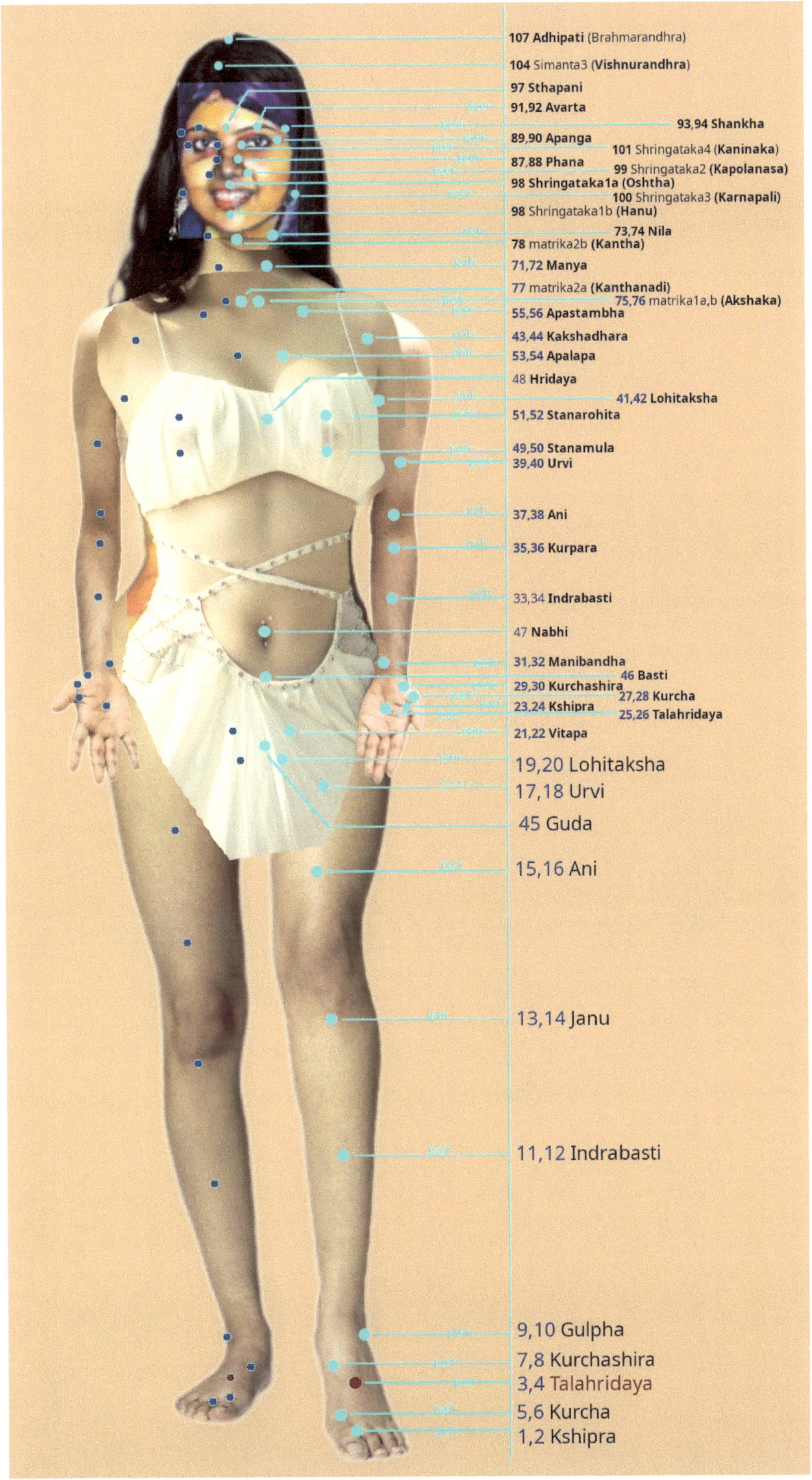

Figure 29 Marma Points Whole Body (Front View – Points of Back are not here)

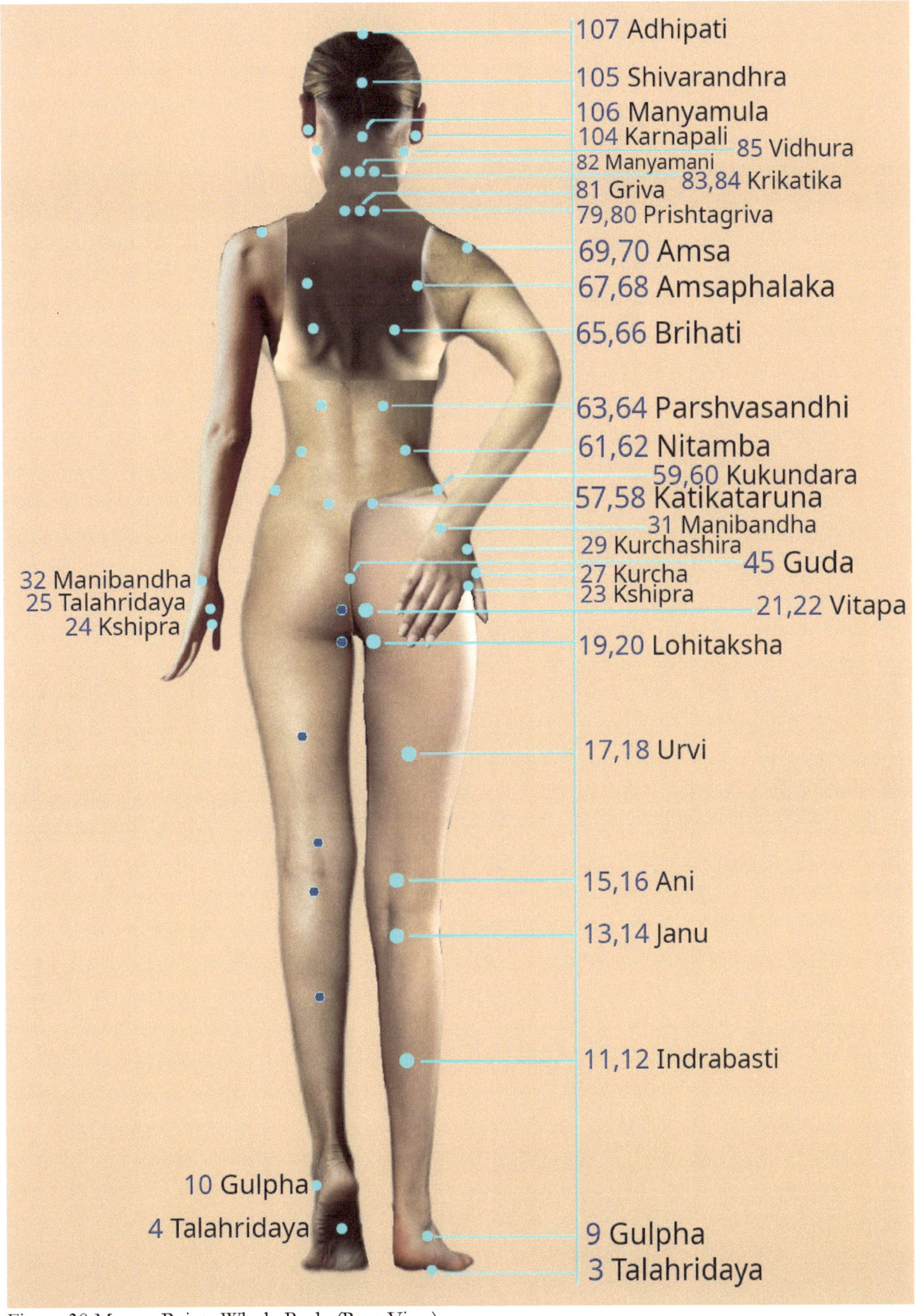

Figure 30 Marma Points Whole Body (Rear View)

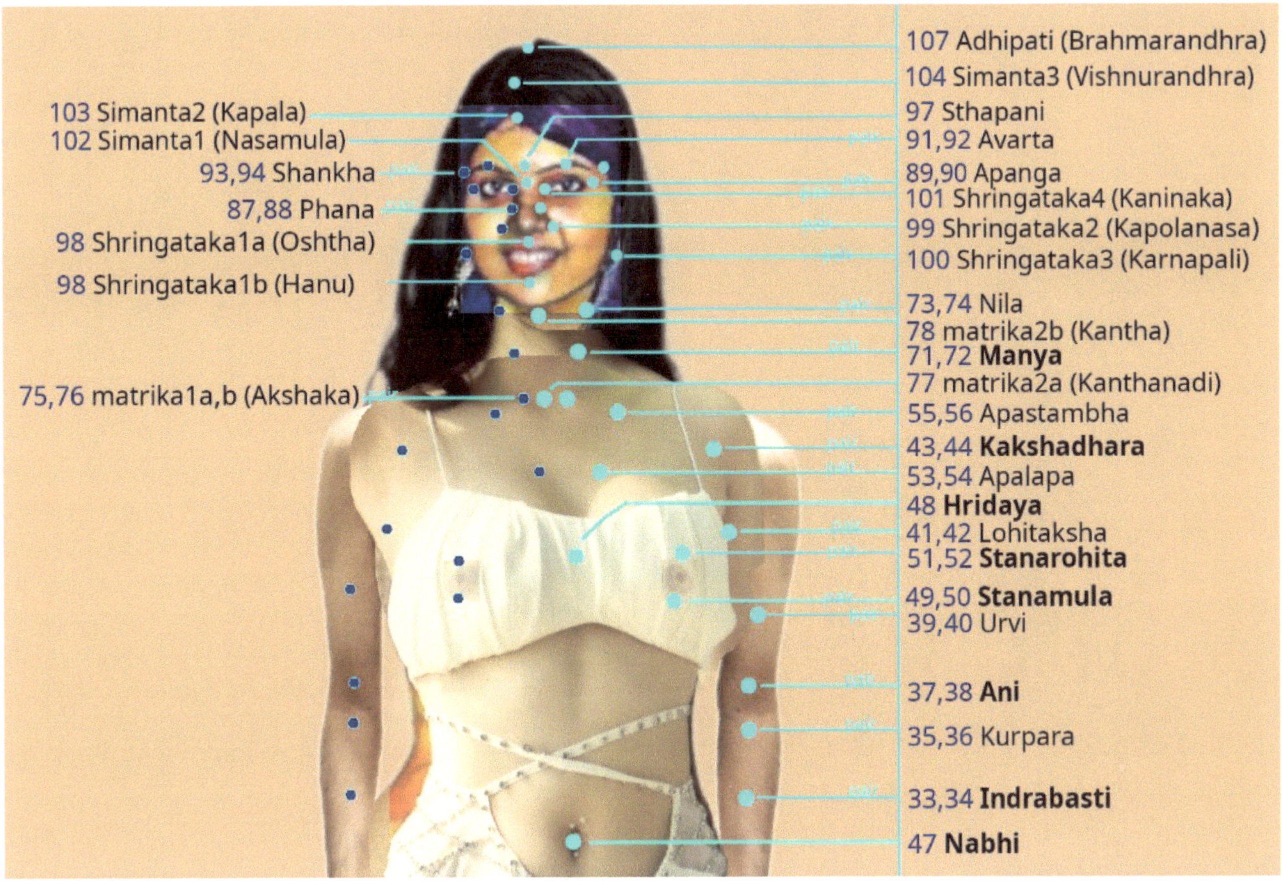

Figure 31 Marma Points Whole Body Front View (Upper Half)

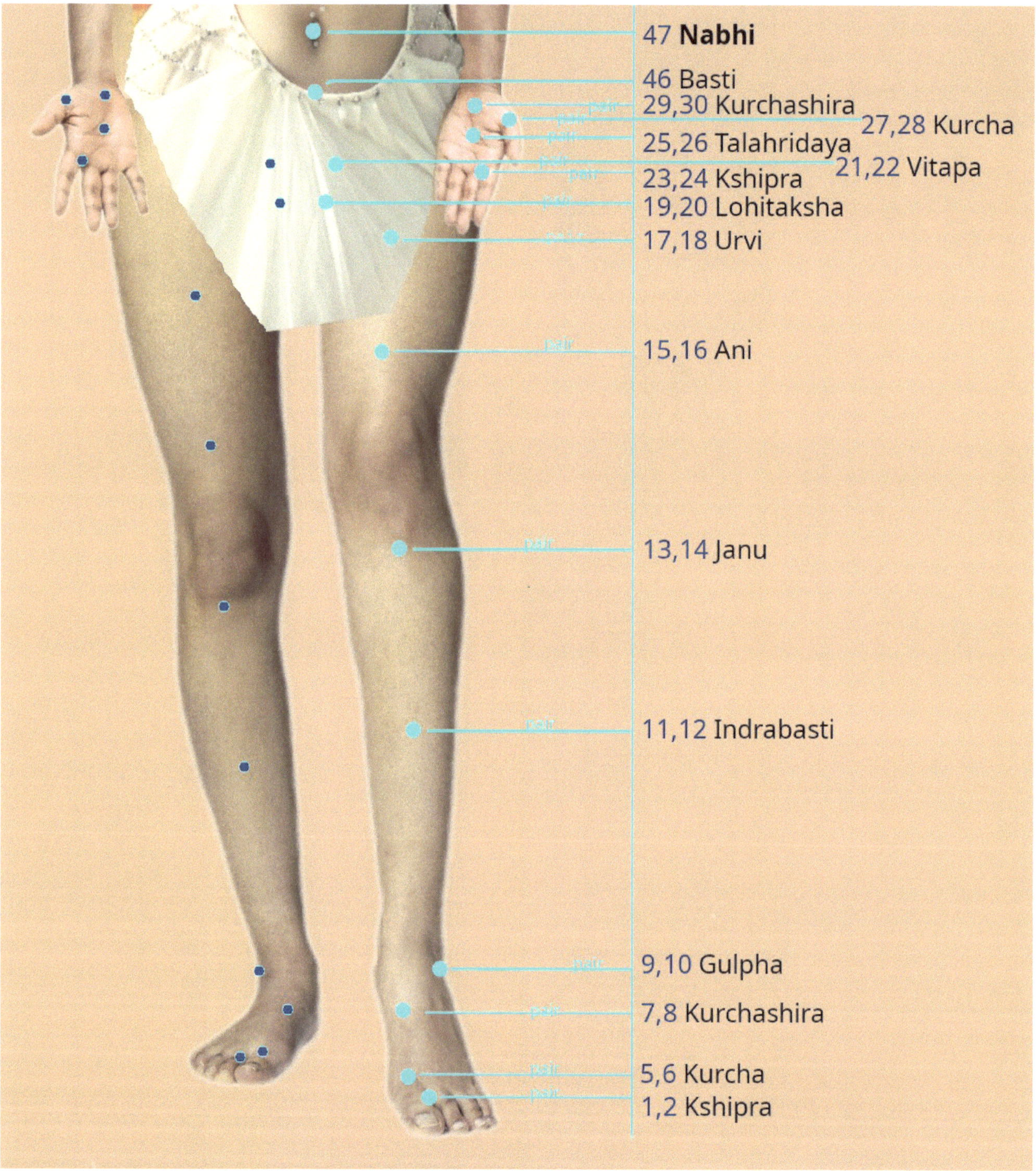

Figure 32 Marma Points Whole Body Front View (Lower Half)

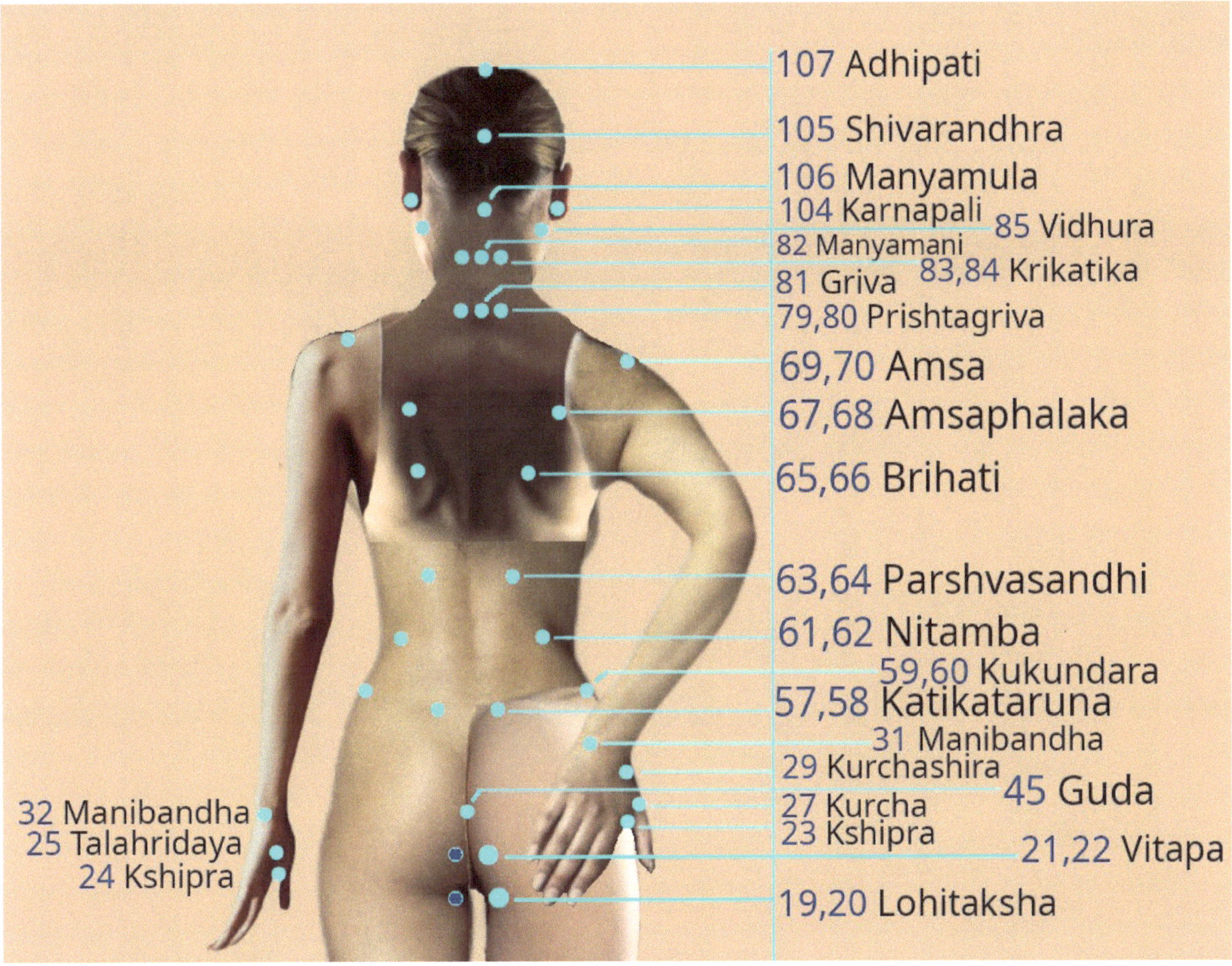

Figure 33 Marma Points Whole Body Rear View (Upper Half)

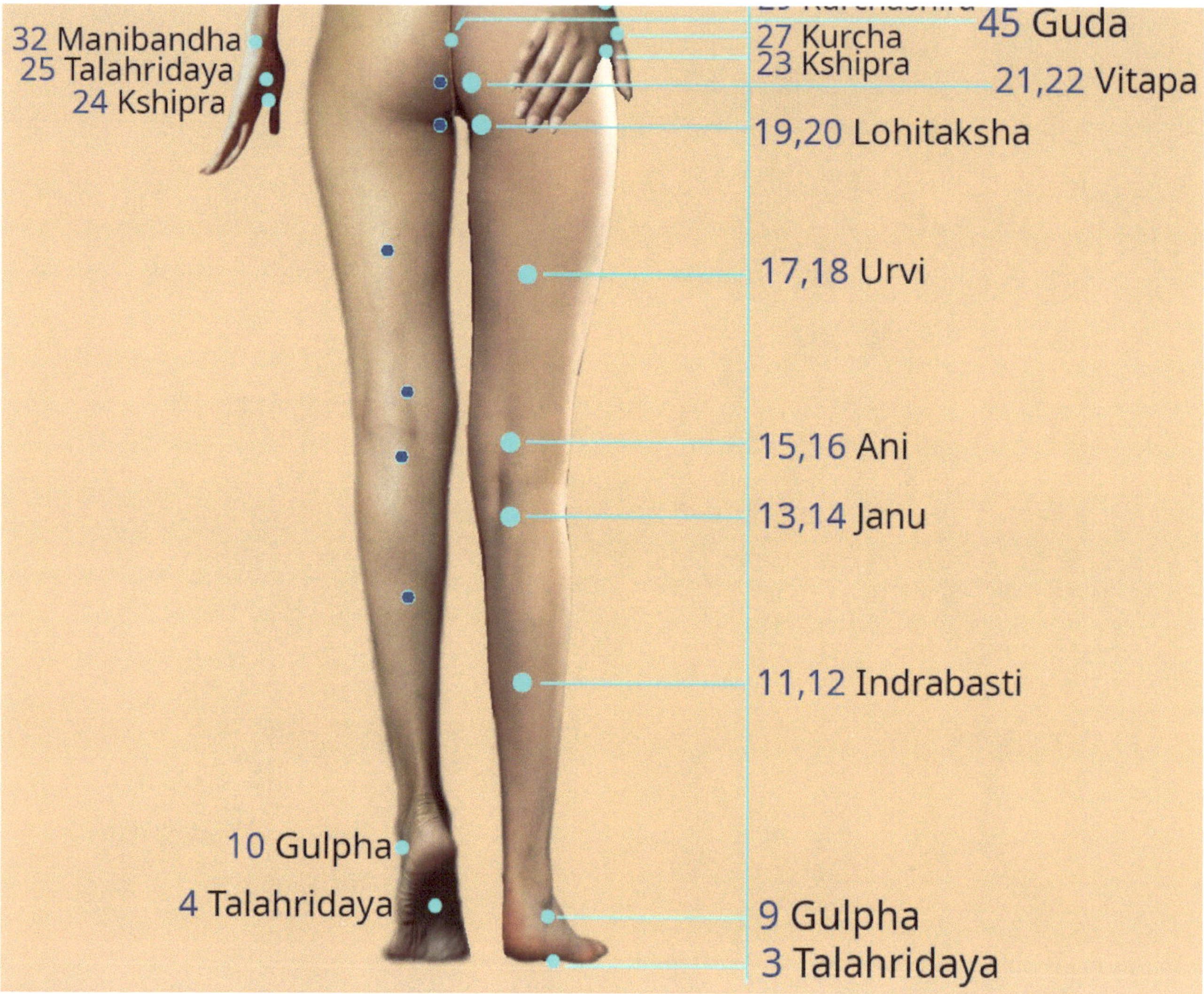

Figure 34 Marma Points Whole Body Rear View (Lower Half)

Ashtanga Hridayam of Vagbhatta - Marma Verses

The classic commentator on Medicine and Surgery of rishis Sushruta and Charaka is named Vagbhatta, and his text called Ashtanga Hridayam consists of 6 Books. 1st SutraSthanam, 2nd ShariraSthanam, 3rd NidanaSthanam, 4th ChikitsaSthanam, 5th KalpaSiddhiSthanam, 6th UttaraSthanam.

The 2nd Book **शारीरस्थानम्** Sharira Sthanam, which is a discussion and description of Human Anatomy, contains the 4th chapter on Marma.

Ashtanga to signify Ayurveda's eight branches, which include:
1. Kaaya Chikitsa – Internal Medicine
2. Baala Chikitsa – Pediatrics
3. Bhuta Vidya – Psychiatry
4. Shalakya Tantra – Ear, Nose and Throat Treatment
5. Shalya Tantra – Surgery
6. Vishagara Vairodh Tantra – Toxicology
7. Jarachikitsa/Rasayana – Geriatrics and Rejuvenation
8. Vajikarana — Aphrodisiac Therapy, Fertility, and Conception

श्रीमद् वाग्भटः विरचितम् अष्टाङ्ग-हृदयम् ॥
स्थानम् – २. शारीरस्थानम् - चतुर्थोऽध्यायः - मर्मविभागशारीरोऽध्यायः ॥
Honorable Vagbhata written Ashtanga Hridayam.
Section – 2. Human Anatomy – 4th Chapter Marma.

अथातो मर्मविभागं शारीरं व्याख्यास्यामः। इति ह स्माहुरात्रेयादयो महर्षयः।
सप्तोत्तरं मर्मशतम् तेषामेकादशादिशेत् । पृथक्सक्थ्नोस्तथा बाह्वोस्त्रीणि कोष्ठे नवोरसि।।१।।
पृष्ठे चतुर्दशोर्ध्वं तु जत्रोस्त्रिंशच्च सप्त च। मध्ये पादतलस्याहुरभितो मध्यमाङ्गुलिम्।।२।।
तलहृन्नाम रुजया तत्र विद्धस्य पञ्चता। अङ्गुष्ठाङ्गुलिमध्यस्थं क्षिप्रमाक्षेपमारणम्।।३।।
तस्योर्ध्वं द्व्यङ्गुले कूर्चः पादभ्रमणकम्पकृत्। गुल्फसन्धेरधः कूर्चशिरःशोफरुजाकरम्।।४।।
जङ्घाचरणयोः सन्धौ गुल्फो रुक्स्तम्भमान्द्यकृत्। जङ्घान्तरे त्विन्द्रबस्तिर्मारयत्यसृजः क्षयात्।।५।।
जङ्घ्घोर्वोः सङ्गमे जानु खञ्जता तत्र जीवतः। जानुनस्त्र्यङ्गुलादूर्ध्वमाण्यूस्तम्भशोफकृत्।।६।।
उर्व्यूरुमध्ये तद्वेधात्सक्थिशोषोऽस्रसङ्क्षयात्। ऊरुमूले लोहिताक्षं हन्ति पक्षमसृक्क्षयात्।।७।।
मुष्कवङ्क्षणयोर्मध्ये विटपं षण्ढताकरम्। इति सक्थ्नोस्तथा बाह्वोर्मणिबन्धोऽत्र गुल्फवत्।।८।।
कूर्परं जानुवत्कौण्यं तयोर्विटपवत्पुनः। कक्षाक्षमध्ये कक्षाधृक् कुणित्वं तत्र जायते।।९।।
इति शाखासु मर्माणि चतुश्चत्वारिंशदुक्त्वा, अन्तराधौ कथयति ----

अधुना बस्त्याख्यमाह-

स्थूलान्त्रबद्धः सद्योघ्नो विड्वातवमनो गुदः। मूत्राशयो धनुर्वक्रो बस्तिरल्पास्रमांसगः।।१०।।
एकाधोवदनो मध्ये कट्याः सद्यो निहन्त्यसून्। ऋतेऽश्मरीव्रणाद्विद्धस्तत्राप्युभयतश्च सः।।११।।
मूत्रस्राव्येकतो भिन्ने व्रणो रोहेच्च यत्नतः। देहामपक्वस्थानानां मध्ये सर्वसिराश्रयः।।१२।।
नाभिः सोऽपि हि सद्योघ्नो---

द्वारमामाशयस्य च। सत्वादिधाम हृदयम् स्तनोरः कोष्ठमध्यगम्।।१३।।
स्तनरोहितमूलाख्ये द्व्यङ्गुले स्तनयोर्वदेत्। ऊर्ध्वाधोऽस्रकफापूर्णकोष्ठो नश्येत्तयोःक्रमात्।।१४।।
अपस्तम्भावुरःपार्श्वे नाड्यावनिलवाहिनी। रक्तेन पूर्णकोष्ठोऽत्र श्वासात्कासाच्च नश्यति।।१५।।
पृष्ठवंशोरसोर्मध्ये तयोरेव च पार्श्वयोः। अधोंऽसकूटयोर्विद्यादपालापाख्यममर्मणी।।१६।। अपस्तम्भौ ??
तयोः कोष्ठेऽसृजा पूर्णे नश्येद्यातेन पूयताम्।
इदानीं पृष्ठे वक्ति----
पार्श्वयोः पृष्ठवंशस्य श्रोणीकर्णौ प्रति स्थिते।।१७।।
वंशाश्रिते स्फिजोरूर्ध्वं कटीकतरुणो स्मृते। तत्र रक्तक्षयात्पाण्डुर्हीनरूपो विनश्यति।।१८।।
पृष्ठवंशं ह्युभयतो यौ सन्धी कटीपार्श्वयोः। जघनस्य बहिर्भागे मर्मणी तौ कुकुन्दरौ।।१९।।
चेष्टाहानिरघःकाये स्पर्शाज्ञानं च तद्व्यधात्। पार्श्वान्तरनिबद्धौ यावुपरि श्रोणिकर्णयोः।।२०।।
आशयच्चादनौ तौ तु नितम्बौ तरुणास्थिगौ। अधःशरीरे शोफोऽत्र दौर्बल्यं मरणं ततः।।२१।।
पार्श्वान्तरनिबद्धौ च मध्ये जघनपार्श्वयोः। तिर्यगूर्ध्वं च निर्दिष्टौ पार्श्वसन्धी तयोर्यधात्।।२२।।
रक्तपूरितकोष्ठस्य शरीरान्तरसम्भवः। स्तनमूलार्जवे भागे पृष्ठवंशाश्रये सिरे।।२३।।
बृहत्यौ, तत्र विद्धस्य मरणं रक्तसङ्क्षयात्। बाहुमूलाभिसम्बद्धे पृष्ठवंशस्य पार्श्वयोः।।२४।।
अंसयोः फलके बाहुस्वापशोषौ तयोर्व्यधात्। ग्रीवामुभयतः स्नाव्नी ग्रीवाबाहुशिरोन्तरे।।२५।।
स्कन्धांसपीठसम्बन्धावंसौ बाहुक्रियाहरौ। कण्ठनाडीमुभयतः सिरा हनुसमाश्रिताः।।२६।।
चतस्रस्तासु नीले द्वे मन्ये द्वे मर्मणी स्मृते। स्वरप्रणाशवकृत्यं रसाज्ञानं च तद्व्यधे।।२७।।
कण्ठनाडीमुभयतो जिह्वानासागताः सिराः। पृथक् चतस्रस्ताः सद्यो घ्नन्त्यसून्मातृकाह्वयाः।।२८।।
कृकाटिके शिरोग्रीवासन्धौ, तत्र चलं शिरः। अधस्तात्कर्णयोर्निम्ने विधुरे श्रुतिहारिणी।।२९।।
फणावुभयतो घ्राणमार्गं श्रोत्रपथानुगौ। अन्तर्गलस्थितौ वेधाद्गन्धविज्ञानहारिणौ।।३०।।
नेत्रयोर्बाह्यतोऽपाङ्गौ भ्रुवोः पुच्छान्तयोरधः। तथोपरि भ्रुवोर्निम्नावावर्तावान्व्यमेषु तु।।३१।।
अनुकर्णं ललाटान्ते शङ्खौ सद्योविनाशनौ। केशान्ते शङ्खयोरूर्ध्वमुत्क्षेपौ, स्थपनी पुनः।।३२।।
भ्रुवोर्मध्ये, त्रयेऽप्यत्र शल्ये जीवेदनुद्धृते। स्वयं वा पतिते पाकात्सद्यो नश्यति तूद्धृते।।३३।।
जिह्वाक्षिनासिकाश्रोत्रखचतुष्टयसङ्गमे। तालुन्यास्यानि चत्वारि स्रोतसां, तेषु मर्मसु।।३४।।
विद्धः शृङ्गाटकाख्येषु सद्यस्त्यजति जीवितम्। कपाले सन्धयः पञ्च सीमन्तास्तिर्यगूर्ध्वगाः।।३५।।
भ्रमोन्मादमनोनाशैस्तेषु विद्धेषु नश्यति। आन्तरो मस्तकस्योर्ध्वं सिरासन्धिसमागमः।।३६।।
रोमावर्तोऽधिपो नाम मर्म सद्यो हरत्यसून्।
इति सप्तोत्तरस्य मर्मशतस्य लक्षणान्युक्त्वा, सामान्येन यन्मर्मलक्षणं तदाख्यातुमाह----
विषमं स्पन्दनं यत्र पीडिते रुक् च मर्म तत्।।३७।।
मांसास्थिस्नायुधमनीसिरासन्धिसमागमः। स्यान्मर्मेति च तेनात्र सुतरां जीवितं स्थितम्।।३८।।
बाहुल्येन तु निर्देशः षोढैवं मर्मकल्पना। प्राणायतनसामान्यदैक्यं वा मर्मणां मतम्।।३९।।
मांसादीनां सन्ध्यन्तानां यथास्वं प्रतिनियतनि मर्माणि सङ्ख्याऽभिधातुमाह ----
मांसजानि दशेन्द्राख्यतलहृत्स्तनरोहिताः। शङ्खौ कटीकतरुणे नितम्बावंसयोः फले।।४०।।
अस्थ्यष्टौ--। स्नावमर्माणि त्रयोविंशतिराणयः। कूर्चकूर्चशिरोऽपाङ्गक्षिप्रोत्क्षेपांसबस्तयः।।४१।।
गुदापस्तम्भविधुरशृङ्गाटानि नवादिशेत्।

मर्माणि धमनीस्थानि— सप्तत्रिंशत्सिराश्रयाः।।४२।।
बृहत्यौ मातृका नीले मन्ये कक्षाधरौ फणौ। विटपे हृदयं नाभिः पार्श्वसन्धी स्तनाधरे।।४३।।
अपालापौ स्थपन्युर्व्यश्चतस्रो लोहितानि च। सन्धौ विंशतिरावर्तौ मणिबन्धौ कुकुन्दरौ।।४४।।
सीमन्ताः कूर्परौ गुल्फौ कृकाट्यौ जानुनी पतिः। मांसमर्म गुदोऽन्येषां,स्नान्नि कक्षाधरौ तथा।।४५।।
विटपौ विधुराख्ये च, शृङ्गाटानि सिरासु तु। अपस्तम्भावपाङ्गौ च, धमनीस्थं न तैः स्मृतम्।।४६।।
इदानीं मांसादिजानां मर्मणां व्यधलक्षणमाह ----
विद्धेऽजस्रमसृक्स्रावो मांसधावनवत्तनुः। पाण्डुत्वमिन्द्रियाज्ञानं मरणं चाशु मांसजे।।४७।।
मज्जान्वितोऽच्छो विच्छिन्नः स्रावो रुक् चास्थिमर्मणी। आयामाक्षेपकस्तम्भाः स्नावजेऽभ्यधिकं रुजा।।४८।।
यानस्थानासनाशक्तिर्वैकल्यमथवाऽन्तकः। रक्तं सशब्दफेनोष्णं धमनीस्थे विचेतसः।।४९।।
सिरामर्मव्यधे सान्द्रमजस्रं बह्वसृक्स्रवेत्। तत्क्षयात्तृड्भ्रमश्वाससमोहहिध्माभिरन्तकः।।५०।।
वस्तु शूकैरिवाकीर्णं रूढे च कुणिखञ्जता। बलचेष्टाक्षयः शोषः पर्वशोफश्च सन्धिजे।।५१।।
नाभिशङ्खाधिपापानहृच्छृङ्गाटकबस्तयः। आष्टौ च मातृकाः सद्यो निघ्नत्येकान्नविंशतिः।।५२।।
सप्ताहः परमस्तेषां कालः कालस्य कर्षणे। त्रयस्त्रिंशदपस्तम्भतलहृत्पार्श्वसन्धयः।।५३।।
कटीतरुणसीमन्तस्तनमूलेन्द्रबस्तयः। क्षिप्रापालापबृहतीनितम्बस्तनरोहिताः।।५४।।
कालान्तरप्राणहरा मासमासार्द्धजीविताः। उत्क्षेपौ स्थपनी त्रीणि विशल्यघ्नानि, तत्र हि।।५५।।
वायुर्मांसवसामज्जमस्तुलुङ्गानि शोषयन्। शल्यापाये विनिर्गच्छन् श्वासात्कासाच्च हन्त्यसून्।।५६।।
फणावपाङ्गौ विधुरे नीले मन्ये कृकाटिके। अंसांसफलकावर्तविटपोर्वीकुकुन्दराः।।५७।।
सजानुलोहिताक्षाणिकक्षाधृक्कूर्चकूर्पराः। वैकल्यमिति चत्वारि चत्वारिंशच्च कुर्वते।।५८।।
हरन्ति तान्यपि प्राणान् कदाचिदभिघाततः। अष्टौ कूर्चशिरोगुल्फमणिबन्धा रुजाकराः।।५९।।
तेषां विटपकक्षाधृगुर्व्यः कूर्चशिरांसि च। द्वादशाङ्गुलमानानि --
द्व्यङ्गुले मणिबन्धने।।६०।। गुल्फौ च स्तनमूले च --
त्र्यङ्गुलं जानुकूर्परम्। अपानबस्तिहृन्नाभिनीलाः सीमन्तमातृकाः।।६१।।
कूर्चश्रृङ्गाटमन्याश्च त्रिंशदेकेन वर्जिताः। आत्मपाणितलोन्मानाः --
शेषाण्यर्द्धाङ्गुलं वदेत्।।६२।। पञ्चाशत्षट् च मर्माणि, तिलव्रीहिसमान्यपि।
इष्टानि मर्माण्यन्येषाम्----इदानीं यथा मर्माभिघाते मरणं सम्पद्यते तथा दर्शयति----
चतुर्द्धोक्ताः सिरास्तु याः।।६३।।
तर्पयन्ति वपुः कृत्स्नं ता मर्माण्याश्रितास्ततः। तत्क्षतात्क्षतजात्यर्थप्रवृत्तेर्धातुसङ्क्षये।।६४।।
वृद्धश्चलो रुजस्तीव्राः प्रतनोति समीरयन्। तेजस्तदुद्धूतं धत्ते तृष्णाशोषमदभ्रमान्।।६५।।
स्विन्नस्रस्तश्लथतनुं हरत्येनं ततोऽन्तकः। वर्धयेत्सन्धितो गात्रं मर्मण्यभिहते द्रुतम्।।६६।।
छेदनात्सन्धिदेशस्य सङ्कुचन्ति सिरा ह्यतः। जीवितं प्राणिनां तत्र रक्ते तिष्ठति तिष्ठति।।६७।।
तदनेन प्रकारेण मर्माभिघातक्षतान्मरणम्, न त्वमर्माभिघातक्षतात्।
अत इदमाह----सुविक्षतोऽप्यतो जीवेदमर्मणि न मर्मणि। प्राणघातिनि जीवेत्तु कश्चिद्वैद्यगुणेन चेत्।।६८।।
असमग्राभिघाताच्च सोऽपि वैकल्यमश्नुते। तस्मत्क्षारविषाग्न्यादीन् यत्नान्मर्मसु वर्जयेत्।।६९।।
मर्माभिघातः स्वल्पोऽपि प्रायशो बाधतेतराम्। रोगा मर्माश्रयास्तद्वत्प्रक्रान्ता यत्नतोऽपि च।।७०।।
इति श्रीवैद्यपतिसिंहगुप्तसूनुश्रीमद्वाग्भटविरचितायाम् अष्टाङ्गहृदय-संहितायां द्वितीये शारीरस्थाने मर्मविभागो नाम चतुर्थोऽध्यायः।।

Here ends the 4th Chapter named the Marma Section of the 2nd book titled Sharira Sthana of Ashtanga Hridayam.

Charaka Samhita - Marma Verses

The Charaka Samhita is a fundamental Medical text on Diagnosis and Healing. It consists of:
I. Sutra Sthanam = Section on fundamental principles
II. Nidana Sthanam = Section on diagnostic principles
III. Vimana Sthanam = Section on specific medical principles
IV. Sharira Sthanam = Section on human being and genesis
V. Indriya Sthanam = Section on sensorial prognosis
VI. Chikitsa Sthanam = Section on therapeutic principles
VII. Kalpa Sthanam = Section on pharmaceutical preparations
VIII. Siddhi Sthanam = Section on therapeutic procedures

Within the सिद्धिस्थानम् Siddhi Sthana ९. त्रिमर्मीया सिद्धिः Chapter 9 Tri Marmiya Siddhi. Verses 1 to 10. These verses give the Marma Points and their attributes in brief.

अथातस्त्रिमर्मीयां सिद्धिं व्याख्यास्यामः।।१।। इति ह स्माह भगवानात्रेयः।।२।। सप्तोत्तरं मर्मशतमस्मिञ्छरीरे
स्कन्धशाखासमाश्रितमग्निवेशः। तेषामन्यतमपीडायां समधिका पीडा भवति चेतनानिबन्धवैशेष्यात्। तत्र शाखाश्रितेभ्यो मर्मभ्यः
स्कन्धाश्रितानि गरीयांसि शाखानां तदाश्रितत्वात् स्कन्धाश्रितेभ्योऽपि हृद्बस्तिशिरांसि तन्मूलत्वाच्छरीरस्य।।३।। तत्र हृदये दश धमन्यः
प्राणापानौ मनो बुद्धिश्चेतना महाभूतानि च नाभ्यामरा इव प्रतिष्ठितानि शिरसि इन्द्रियाणि इन्द्रियप्राणवहानि च स्रोतांसि सूर्यमिव गभस्तयः
संश्रितानि बस्तिस्तु स्थूलगुदमुष्कसेवनीशुक्रमूत्रवाहिनीनां नाडीनां मध्ये मूत्रधारोऽम्बुवहानां सर्वस्रोतसामुदधिरिवापगानां प्रतिष्ठा बहुभिश्च
तन्मूलैर्मर्मसञ्ज्ञकैः स्रोतोभिर्गगनमिव दिनकरकरैर्व्याप्तमिदं शरीरम्।।४।। तेषां त्रयाणामन्यतमस्यापि भेदादाश्वेव शरीरभेदः स्यात्
आश्रयनाशादाश्रितस्यापि विनाशः तदुपघातात्तु घोरतरव्याधिप्रादुर्भावः तस्मादेतानि विशेषेण रक्ष्याणि बाह्याभिघाद्वातादिभ्यश्च।।५।। तत्र
हृद्यभिहते कासश्वासबलक्षयकण्ठशोषक्लोमाकर्षणजिह्वानिर्गममुखतालुशोषापस्मारोन्मादप्रलापचित्तनाशादयः स्युः शिरस्यभिहते
मन्यास्तम्भार्दितचक्षुर्विभ्रममोहोद्वेष्टनचेष्टानाशकासश्वासहनुग्रहमूकगद्गदत्वाक्षिनिमीलन-
गण्डस्पन्दनजृम्भणलालास्रावस्वरहानिवदनजिह्मत्वादीनि बस्तौ तु वातमूत्रवर्चोनिग्रहवङ्क्षणमेहनबस्तिशूलकुण्डलोदावर्तगुल्मानिला-
ष्ठीलोपस्तम्भनाभिकुक्षिगुदश्रोणिग्रहादयः वाताद्युपसृष्टानां त्वेषां लिङ्गानि चिकित्सिते सक्रियाविधीन्युक्तानि।।६।। किन्त्वेतानि
विशेषतोऽनिलाद्रक्ष्याणि अनिलो हि पित्तकफसमुदीरणे हेतुः प्राणमूलं च स बस्तिकर्मसाध्यतमः तस्मान्न बस्तिसमं किञ्चित् कर्म
मर्मपरिपालनमस्ति। तत्र षडास्थापनस्कन्धान् विमाने द्वौ चानुवासनस्कन्धाविह च विहितान् बस्तीन् बुध्या विचार्य महामर्मपरिपालनार्थं
प्रयोजयेद्वातव्याधिचिकित्सां च।।७।। भूयश्च हृद्युपसृष्टे हिङ्गुचूर्णं लवणानामन्यतमचूर्णसंयुक्तं मातुलुङ्गस्य रसेनान्येन वाऽम्लेन हृद्येन वा
पाययेत् स्थिरादिपञ्चमूलीरसः सशर्करः पानार्थं बिल्वादिपञ्चमूलरससिद्धा च यवागूः हृद्रोगविहितं च कर्म मूर्ध्नि तु
वातोपसृष्टेऽभ्यङ्गस्वेदनोपनाहस्नेहपाननस्तःकर्मावपीडनधूमादीनि बस्तौ तु कुम्भीस्वेदः वर्तयः श्यामादिभिर्गोमूत्रसिद्धो निरूहः
बिल्वादिभिश्च सुरासिद्धः शरकाशेक्षुदर्भगोक्षुरकमूलश्रृतक्षीरैश्च त्रपुसैर्वारुखराश्वाबीजयवर्षभकवृद्धिकल्कितो निरूहः
पीतदारुसिद्धतैलेनानुवासनं तैल्वकं च सर्पिर्विरेकार्थं शतावरीगोक्षुरकबृहतीकण्टकारिकागुडूचीपुनर्नवोशीरमधुकद्विसारिवालोध्र-
श्रेयसीकुशकाशमूलकषायक्षीरचतुर्गुणं बलावृषर्षभकखराश्वोपकुञ्चिकावत्सकत्रपुसैर्वारुबीजशितिवारकमधुकवचा-
शतपुष्पाश्मभेदकवर्षाभूमदनफलकल्कसिद्धं तैलमुत्तरबस्तिर्निरूहो वा शुद्धस्निग्धस्विन्नस्य बस्तिशूलमूत्रविकारहर इति।।८।।
भवन्ति चात्र श्लोकाः - हृदये मूर्ध्नि बस्तौ च नृणां प्राणाः प्रतिष्ठिताः। तस्मात्तेषां सदा यत्नं कुर्वीत परिपालने।।९।। आबाधवर्जनं नित्यं
स्वस्थवृत्तानुवर्तनम्। उत्पन्नार्तिविघातश्च मर्मणां परिपालनम्।।१०।।

107 Marma Points Alphabetical wrt Body Anatomy

Here we list the Marma Points alphabetically. We also give their location in Anatomy.

S No	Sanskrit Name	No of Points	Body Anatomy Name
1	Adhipati	1	Crown Brahmarandhra
2	Amsaphalaka	2	shoulder blade top
3	Amsa	2	Neck joint backside
4	Ani arm	2	lower part of upper arm frontside
5	Ani leg	2	lower part of upper leg frontside
6	Apalapa	2	upper breast cleavage
7	Apanga	2	outer corner of eye
8	Apastambha	2	directly below clavicle
9	Avarta	2	midpoint above each eye
10	Bahvi / Urvi	2	upper arm midpoint
11	Basti	1	bladder
12	Brihati	2	shoulder blade middle
13	Guda	1	anus
14	Gulpha	2	ankle
15	Hridaya	1	heart
16	Indrabasti arm	2	forearm midpoint
17	Indrabasti leg	2	lower leg midpoint backside
18	Janu	2	knee joint
19	Kakshadhara	2	shoulder joint top
20	Katikataruna	2	hip joint
21	Krikatika	2	neck joint
22	Kshipra hand	2	junction of thumb and index finger
23	Kshipra foot	2	junction of big toe and next toe finger
24	Kukundara	2	lower iliac spine at pelvis
25	Kurcha hand	2	thumb base
26	Kurcha foot	2	big toe base
27	KurchaShira hand	2	tuft of thumb all the way till it extends near wrist
28	KurchaShira foot	2	tuft of big toe all the way till it extends near ankle
29	Kurpara	2	elbow joint
30	Lohitaksha arm	2	lower front end of shoulder joint
31	Lohitaksha leg	2	lower front end of hip joint
32	Manibandha	2	wrist
33	Manya	2	upper throat sides sternocleidomastoid muscle
34	Matrika / SiraMatrika	8	2 Points in throat straight line i.e., neck joins head[1], groove below adam's apple[1] 2 Points on either side of groove[2] 2 Points in neck rear in straight line i.e., neck joins head[1], neck joins torso[1] 2 Points on either side where neck joins torso[2]

35	Nabhi	1	navel
36	Nila	2	side of lower throat sternocleidomastoid muscle
37	Nitamba	2	upper buttocks center
38	Parshvasandhi	2	upper buttocks towards spine
39	Phana	2	nose edge line midpoint
40	Shankha	2	temple
41	Shringataka	4	Nerves related to smell, hearing, sight, taste; 4 pairs shringataka 1a, 1b - Related to Tongue – upper lip **oṣṭha**, chin **hanu** shringataka 2a, 2b - Related to Nostrils - **kapola nāsā** pair shringataka 3a, 3b - Related to Ears - earlobes **karṇapāli** pair shringataka 4a, 4b - Related to Eyes - pupils **kanīnakā** pair
42	Simanta	5	skull fissures Manyamula[5], Shivarandhra[4], Vishnurandhra[3], Kapala[2], NasaMula[1]
43	Stana Mula	2	breast below nipple
44	Stana Rohita	2	breast above nipple
45	Sthapani	1	3rd eye – in between eyebrows
46	Tala Hridaya hand	2	palm center
47	Tala Hridaya foot	2	sole center
48	Utkshepa	2	Above ears
49	Urvi	2	upper thigh midpoint
50	Vidhura	2	Behind ears lower side
51	Vitapa	2	Perineum
Marma Points Total		**107**	

107 Marma Points Anatomical Distribution Head to Toe

For clarity and ease, we group the Marma Points under these arbitrary anatomical heads.

a	Single Points in Midline Vertical Axis of body	(6x1) +1	7
b	Multiple Points in Skull	1x5	5
c	Pair Points in Face	4+(5x2)	14
d	Pair Points in Neck	(8x2) -1	15
e	Pair Points in Chest	4x2	8
f	Pair Points at Back	7x2	14
g	Pair Points at Genitals	2x2	4
h	Pair Points in Arms	7x2	14
i	Pair Points in Hands	4x2	8
j	Pair Points in Legs	5x2	10
k	Pair Points in Feet	4x2	8
	Marma Points Total		**107**
Note: This chart excludes points that have already been accounted for. E.g., Adhipati is accounted for under a), so it is not included again under b)			

Now we give the complete features of each Marma point. The Marma No is an arbitrary number used in this book to help identify on the image.

Discrete Points in Midline Vertical Axis of body = (1x6)+1 = 7

Chakra		Marma Name		Anatomy	Remarks
7th chakra	Sahasrara	Adhipati	1	crown	Brahmarandhra/Mūrdhni मूर्ध्नि
6th chakra	Ajna	Sthapani	1	3rd eye	
4th chakra	Anahata	Hridaya	1	heart	
3rd chakra	Manipura	Nabhi	1	navel	
2nd chakra	Svadisthana	Basti	1	bladder	
1st chakra	Mooladhara	Guda	1	anus	
		subTotal	**6**		
5th chakra	Vishuddhi	Kanthanadi	1	throat groove	1 point out of matrika 4 pairs
		Points subTotal	**7**	Corresponding to the 7 Chakras	

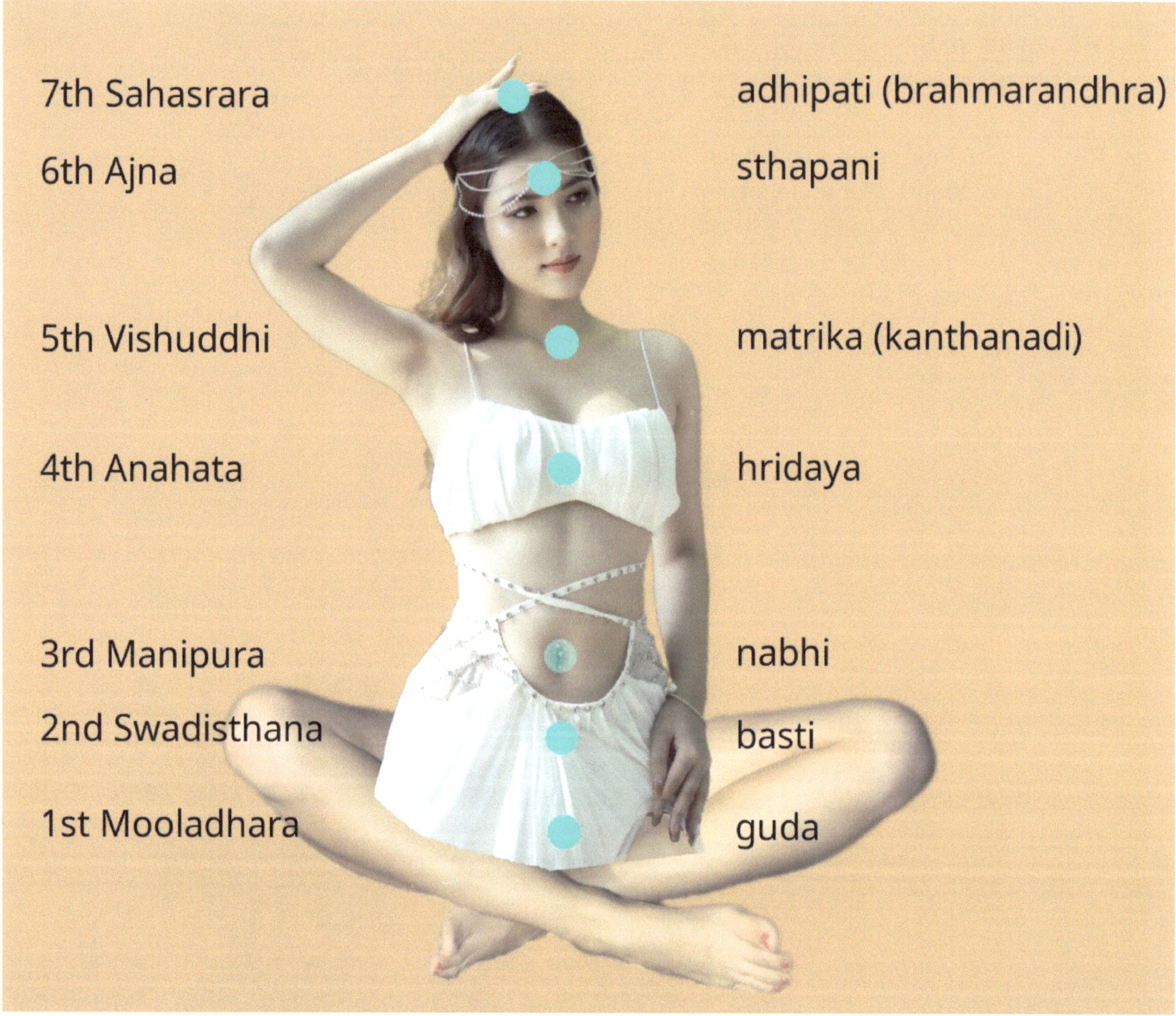

Figure 35: Marma Points Midline Vertical Axis

107. Adhipati (Brahmarandhra) Features

A	Name	अधिपति Adhipati, Brahmarandhra, Murdhni, Sahasrara Chakra
B	Marma No. No of Points	107. One
C	Body Part	Skull
D	Precise Location	Sagittal suture midpoint. Highest point in head.
E	Tissue Type	Sandhi (Joint)
F	Size	½ angula
G	Severity	sadyaḥprāṇaharai = instantly fatal
H	Physics/Chemistry	Sahasrara Chakra. Amygdala. Pineal Gland. Master control.
I	Chikitsa recommended	Touch lightly with Index finger tip. May do a slow roll of fingertip.
J	Oil recommended	Almond. Brahmi. Brahmi Amla. Generous pouring of oil.
K	Meditation / Yogasana	Sudarshan Kriya. Hari Om Meditation.

Adhipati, Sthapani

97. Sthapani Features

A	Name	अधिपति Sthapani, 3rd Eye, Ajna Chakra, 6th chakra
B	Marma No. No of Points	97. One
C	Body Part	Skull
D	Precise Location	In between the eyebrows.
E	Tissue Type	sirā (Tube Vein or Artery)
F	Size	½ angula
G	Severity	viśalyaghna = fatal upon extraction of foreign matter
H	Physics/Chemistry	Pineal Gland. 3rd Eye. Awareness. Master control for entire body mind.
I	Chikitsa recommended	Touch lightly with Index finger tip. May do a slow roll of fingertip.
J	Oil recommended	A2 Ghee. Balm.
K	Meditation / Yogasana	Sudarshan Kriya

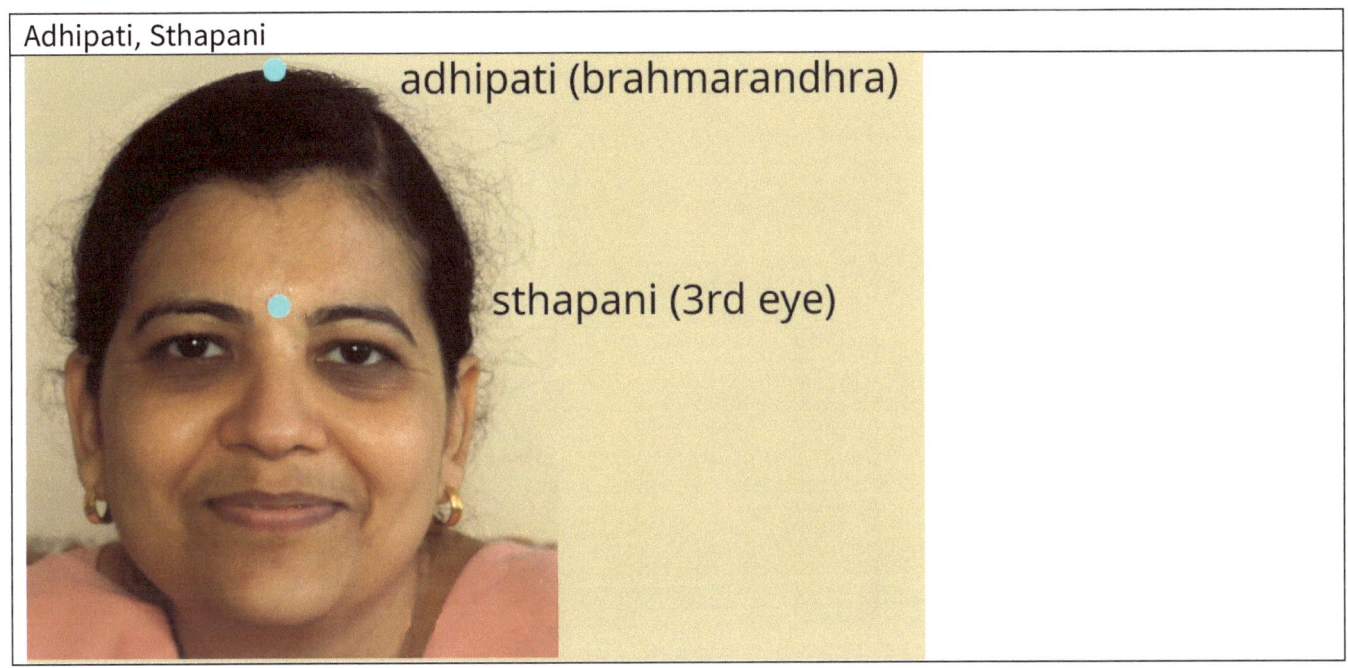

77. Matrika2a (Kanthanadi) Features

A	Name	कण्ठनाडी kaṇṭhanāḍī (kanthanadi)
B	Marma No. No of Points	77. One
C	Body Part	Throat
D	Precise Location	Groove below adam's apple
E	Tissue Type	sirā (Tube Vein or Artery)
F	Size	Palm size
G	Severity	sadyaḥprāṇahara = instantly fatal
H	Physics/Chemistry	Vishuddhi Chakra. Master control for all Communication.
I	Chikitsa recommended	Touch gently with Index finger tip. May do a slow roll of fingertip.
J	Oil recommended	A2 Ghee. Rose Oil.
K	Meditation / Yogasana	Chakra Meditation. Hari Om Meditation. Sudarshan Kriya

kanthanadi, hridaya

48. Hridaya Features

A	Name	हृदय hṛdaya (hridaya)
B	Marma No. No of Points	48. One
C	Body Part	Chest
D	Precise Location	Heart center
E	Tissue Type	sirā (Tube Vein or Artery)
F	Size	Palm size
G	Severity	sadyaḥprāṇahara = instantly fatal
H	Physics/Chemistry	Seat of Soul. Seat of Love.
I	Chikitsa recommended	Press firmly with Index finger tip. May do a slow roll of fingertip.
J	Oil recommended	Fresh Cream. Aloe Vera Gel.
K	Meditation / Yogasana	Sudarshan Kriya

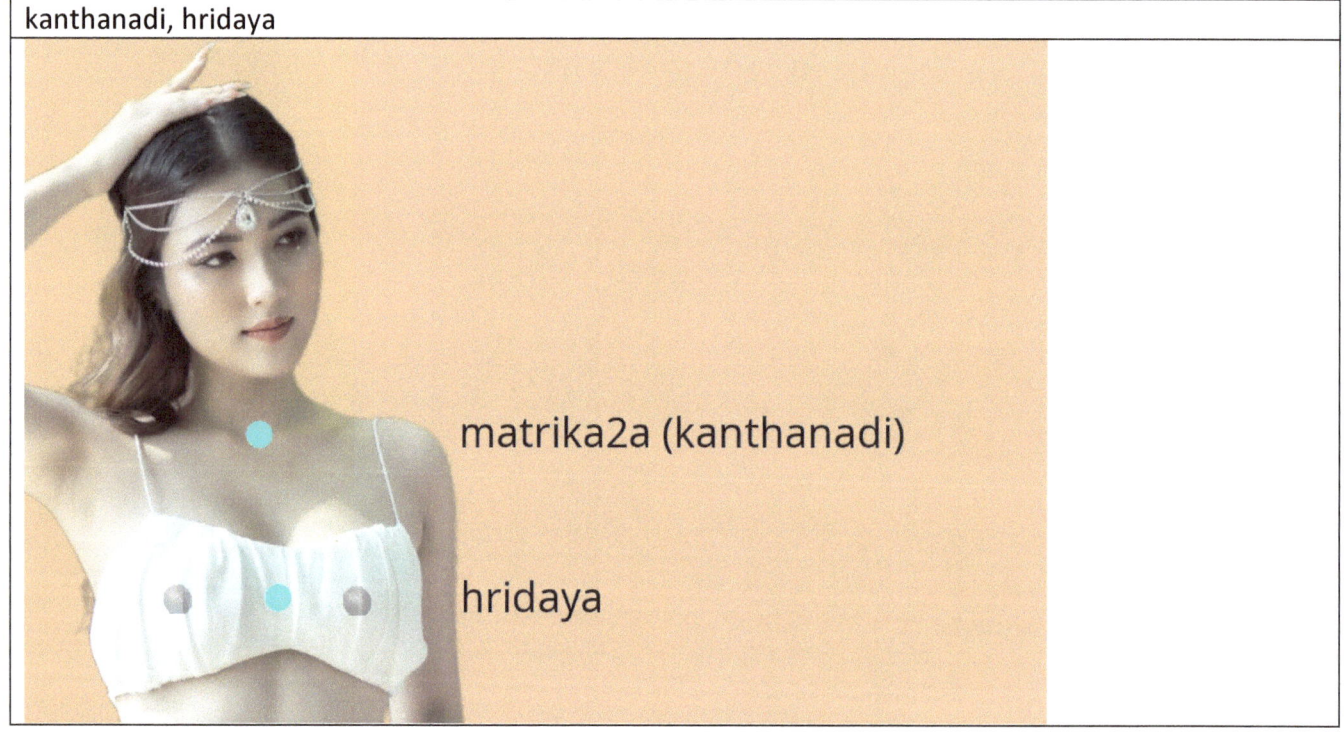

47. Nabhi Features

A	Name	नाभि nābhi (nabhi)
B	Marma No. No of Points	47. One
C	Body Part	Abdomen
D	Precise Location	Navel
E	Tissue Type	sirā (Tube Vein or Artery)
F	Size	Palm size
G	Severity	sadyaḥprāṇahara = instantly fatal
H	Physics/Chemistry	Manipura Chakra. Master control for entire body mind well-being.
I	Chikitsa recommended	Press firmly with Palm just below navel and rock the palm to and fro
J	Oil recommended	A2 Ghee. Dhanwantharam Oil. Use generous amount.
K	Meditation / Yogasana	Chakra Meditation. Hari Om Meditation. Sudarshan Kriya.

nabhi, basti

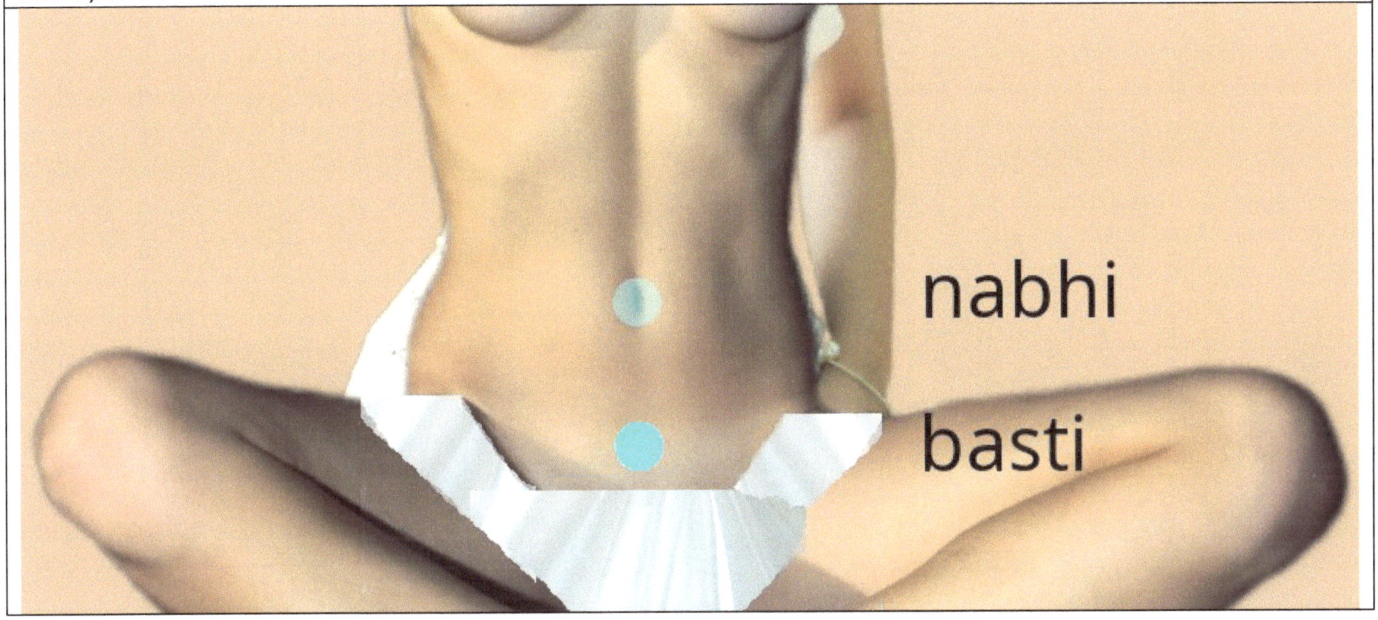

46. Basti Features

A	Name	बस्ति basti
B	Marma No. No of Points	46. One
C	Body Part	Abdomen
D	Precise Location	Bladder, 4 angula below the Navel
E	Tissue Type	snāyu (Nerve/Tendon)
F	Size	Palm size
G	Severity	sadyaḥprāṇahara = instantly fatal
H	Physics/Chemistry	Holding and Storing short term memory.
I	Chikitsa recommended	Press firmly with Index finger tip. May do a slow roll of fingertip.
J	Oil recommended	Dhanwantharam Oil. Use generous amount.
K	Meditation / Yogasana	Hari Om Meditation. Moolabandha. Uddiyana bandha.

45. Guda Features

A	Name	गुद् guda
B	Marma No. No of Points	45. One
C	Body Part	Abdomen
D	Precise Location	anus
E	Tissue Type	māṃsa (Muscle)
F	Size	Palm size
G	Severity	sadyaḥprāṇahara = instantly fatal:
H	Physics/Chemistry	Intuition. Instinct. Awareness.
I	Chikitsa recommended	Palming.
J	Oil recommended	Ashwagandha. Kshirabala.
K	Meditation / Yogasana	Hari Om Meditation. Moolabandha. Ashwini Mudra.

guda

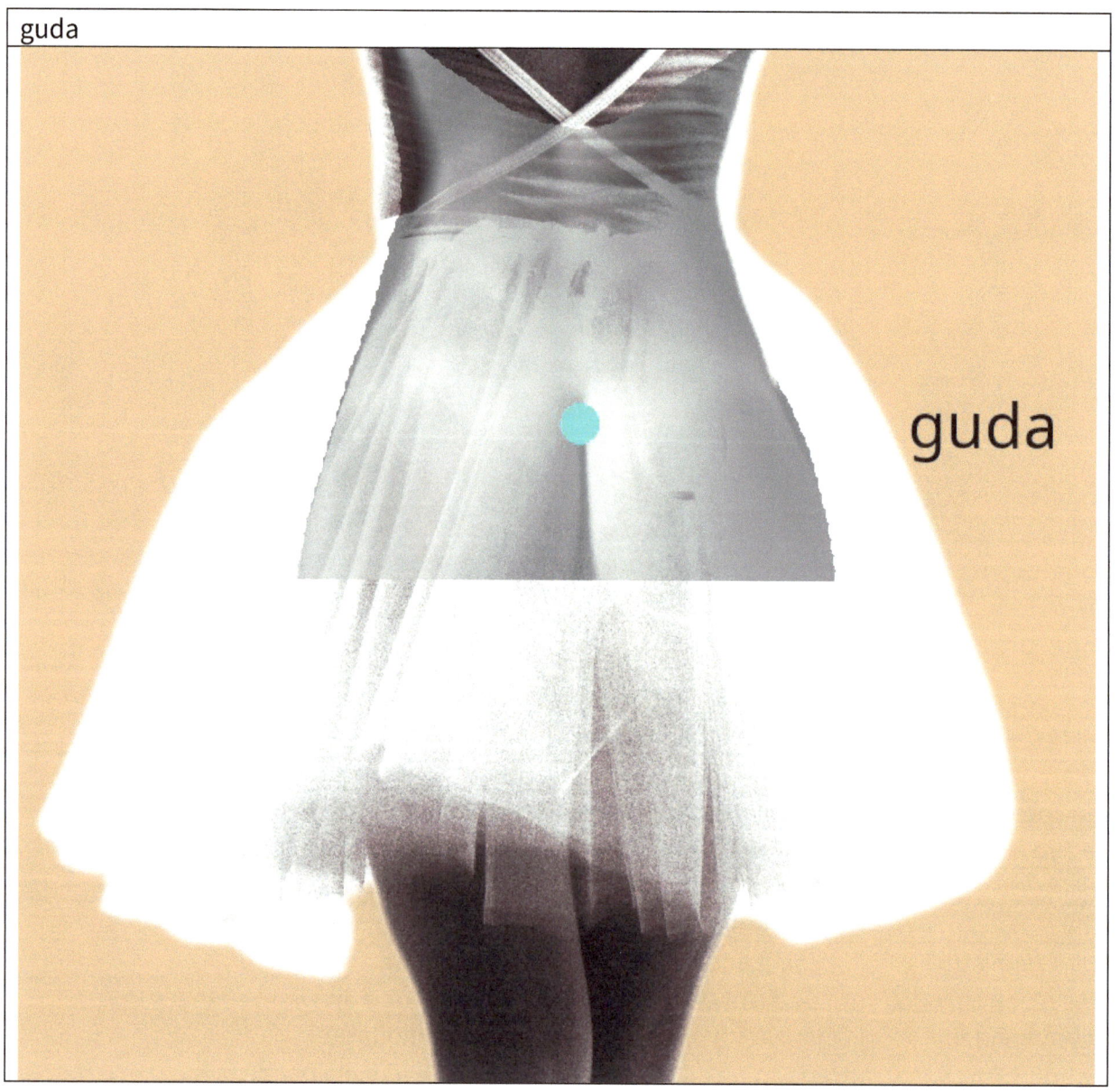

Discrete Points in Skull = 1x5 = 5

Simanta	5	skull fissures / partitions = Nasamula[1], Kapala[2], Vishnurandhra[3], Shivarandhra[4], Manyamula[5]
Points subTotal	**5**	*(and* Adhipati *accounted for earlier)*

Simanta Marma Points
102 = 1. Nasamula is the point at the root of nose at top, just **below** the 3rd eye Sthapani.
103 = 2. Kapala is the point at the hairline on top of the forehead, **above** the 3rd eye Sthapani.
104 = 3. Vishnurandhra (anterior fontanelle) is the point **four angula fore** of Adhipati.
105 = 4. Shivarandhra (posterior fontanelle) is the point known as "choti or shikha शिखा", from where tuft of hair grow and girls make a ponytail. It is **four angula** distance **aft** of Adhipati.
106 = 5. Manyamula is the groove at base of skull at back where the spine starts. It is **in line** with Nasamula if we bisect the head.
107 = Adhipati Marma Point (*has been accounted for earlier*) The **highest** point of the head, **midway** of the sagittal suture. It is also referred to as Brahmarandhra.

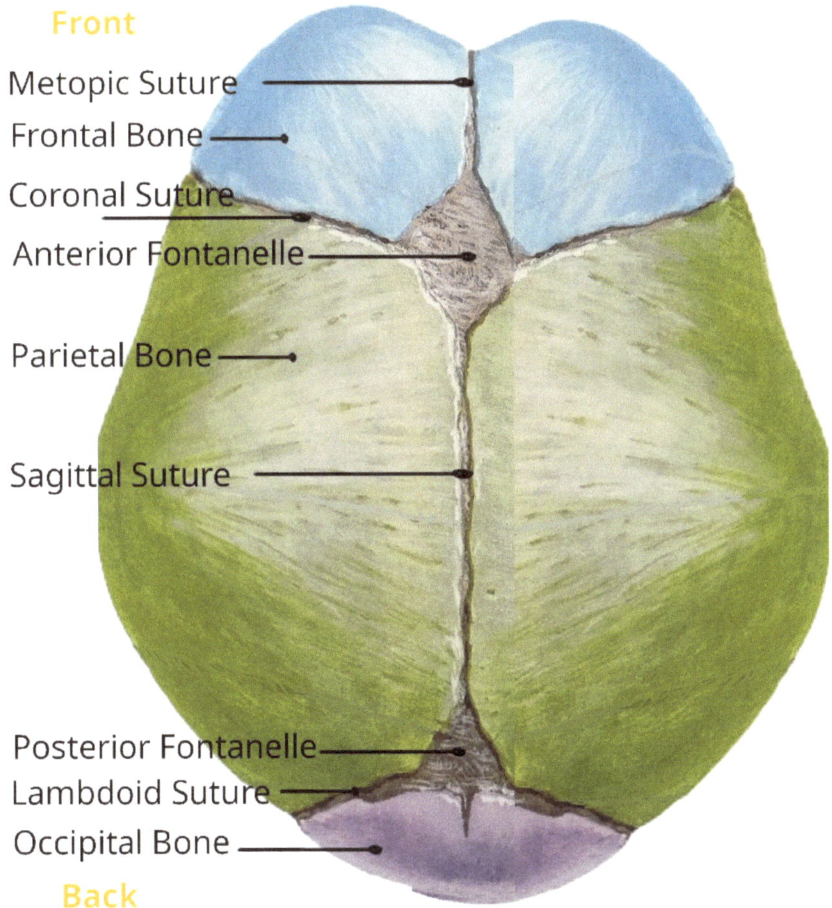

Figure 36: Schematic of Skull (Top View)

Shows 4/5 Simanta Marma Points, and Adhipati

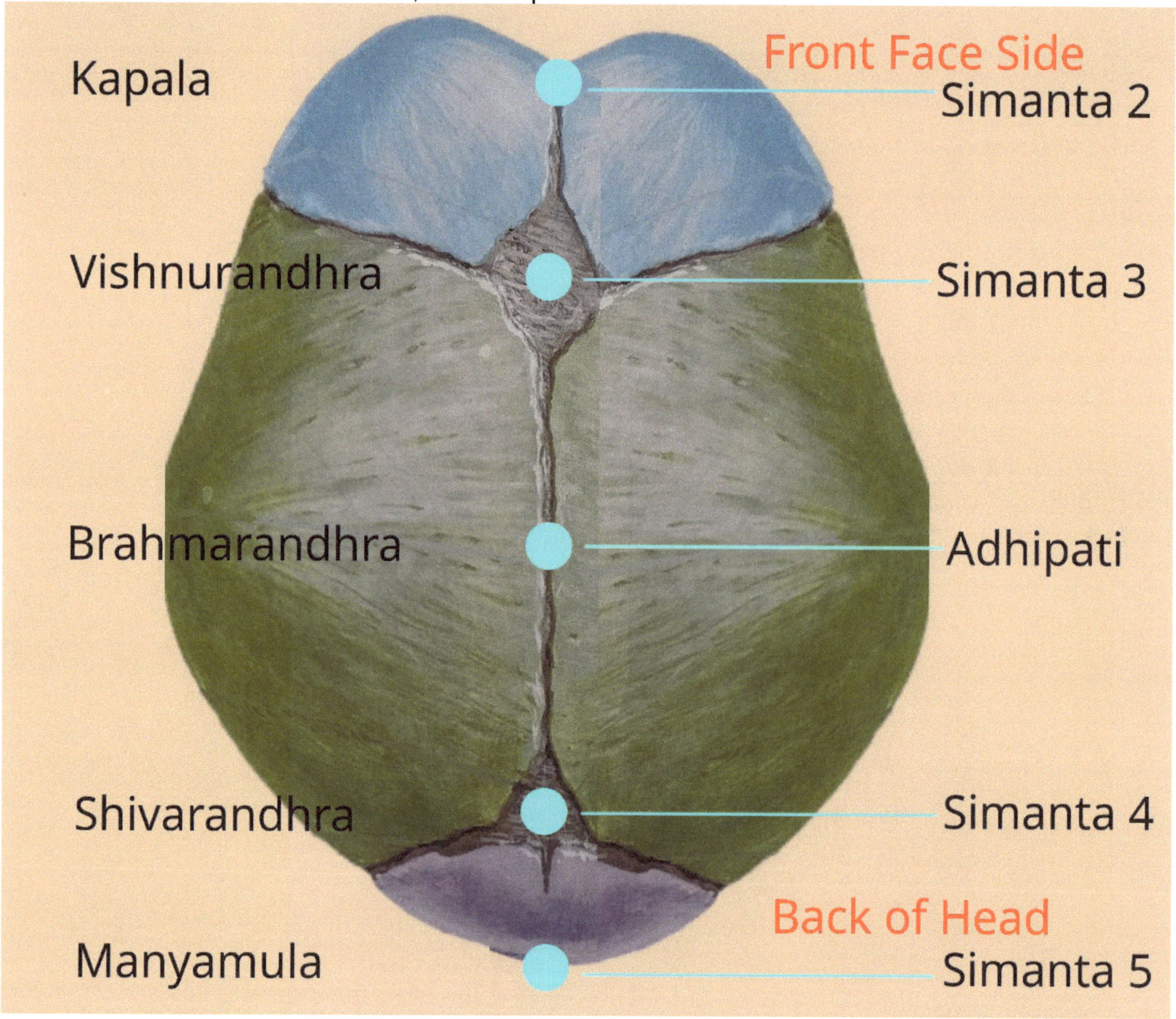

Figure 37: Marma Points in Skull (Top View)

Marma Points in Skull (Back View)
Shows 2/5 Simanta Marma Points (shivarandhra[4], manyamula[5]), and Adhipati

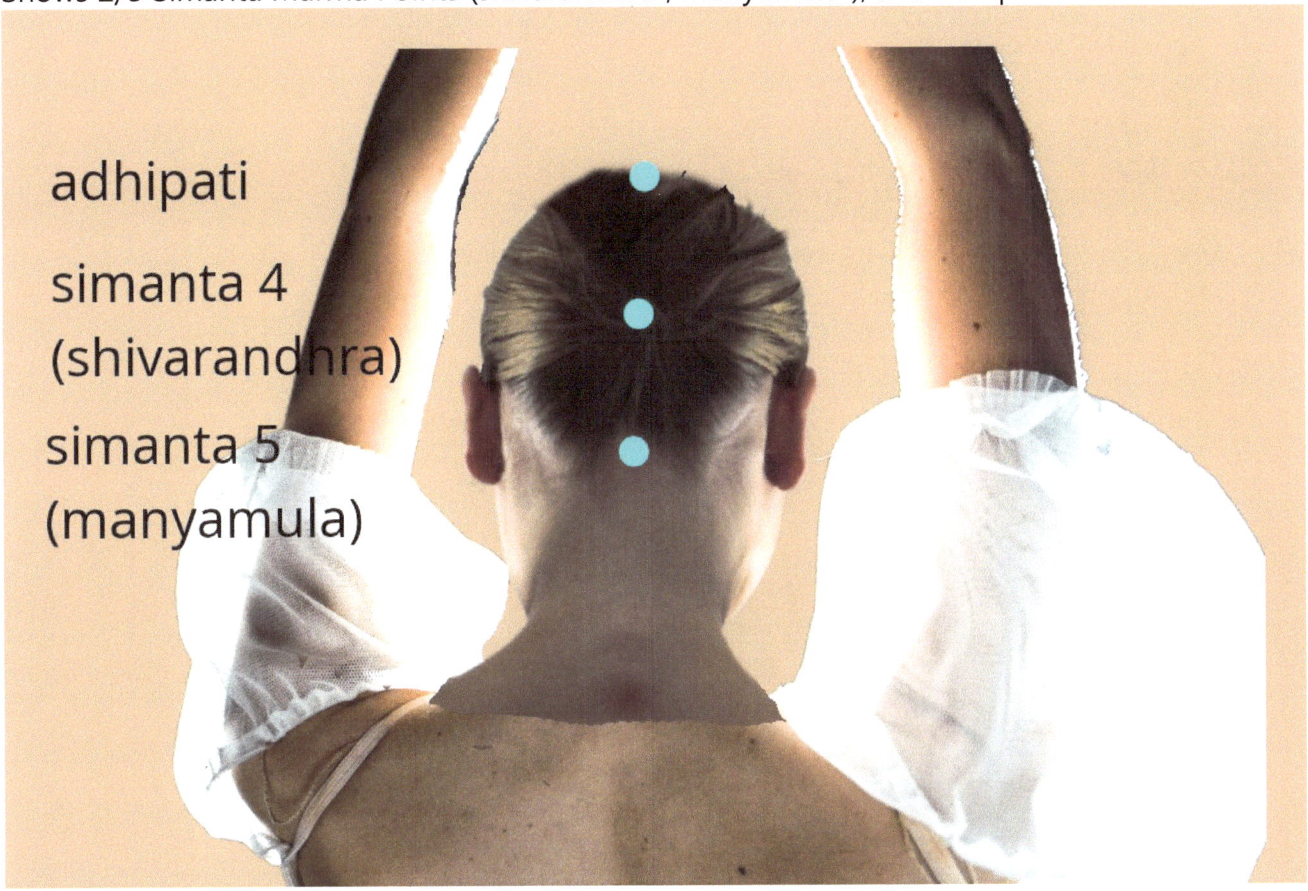

Figure 38: Marma Points in Skull (Back View)

Note:
Typically, the literature refers to the **topmost** area on the skull as the **crown** of the head. Various texts call it the Sahasrara Chakra or the 7th Chakra, and also call it the Brahmarandhra, to mean the **opening** from where the Consciousness enters the body at the time of conception to birth. Since in this book on Marma, the **crown has three distinct Marma points**, we arbitrarily name the points as the triad Brahma-Vishnu-Shiva, i.e., Brahmarandhra-Vishnurandhra-Shivarandhra.

Also, since the literature frequently refers to the opening as Brahmarandhra,

- we name the anterior fontanelle as Vishnurandhra,
- the midway of the sagittal suture as Brahmarandhra, and
- the posterior fontanelle as Shivarandhra.

106. Simanta5 (Manyamula) Features

A	Name	मन्यामूल manyāmūla (manyamula)
B	Marma No. No of Points	106. One
C	Body Part	Skull
D	Precise Location	Posterior fontanelle. Inline with ears the groove at rear of head
E	Tissue Type	sandhi (Joint)
F	Size	Palm size
G	Severity	kālāntaraprāṇahara = fatal after a while
H	Physics/Chemistry	Hypothalamus / Intuition. Instinct. Awareness.
I	Chikitsa recommended	Touch firmly with Index finger tip. May do a slow roll of fingertip.
J	Oil recommended	Brahmi. Brahmi Amla. Almond. Generous pouring of oil.
K	Meditation / Yogasana	Gurudev's Guided Meditation. Sudarshan Kriya.

manyamula, shivarandhra

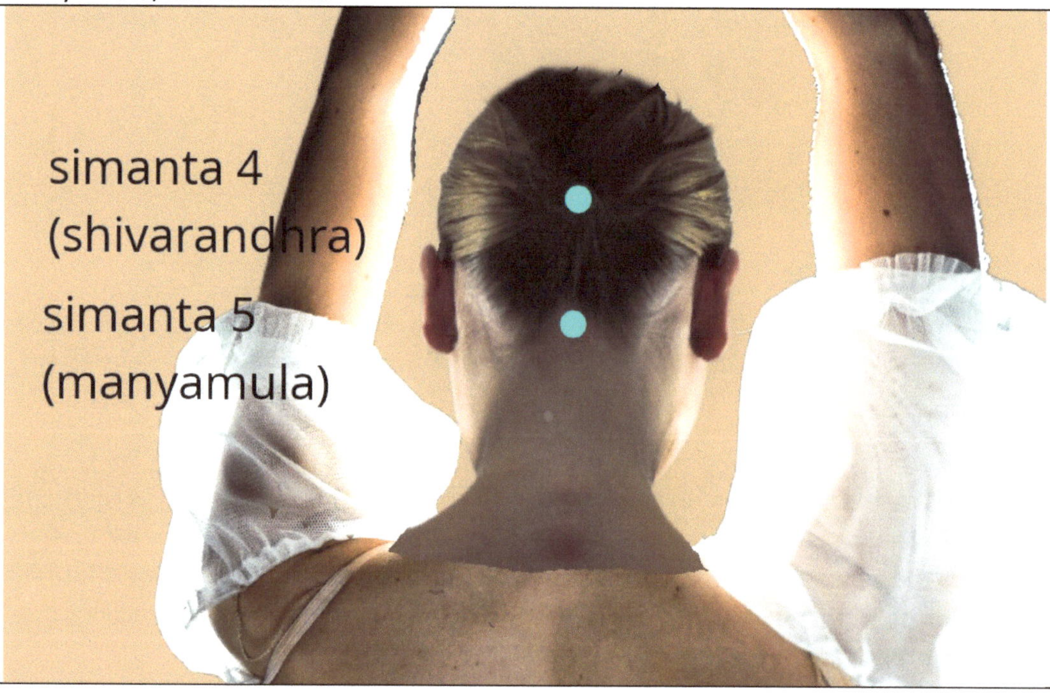

105. Simanta4 (Shivarandhra) Features

A	Name	शिवरन्ध्र śivarandhra (shivarandhra)
B	Marma No. No of Points	105. One
C	Body Part	Skull
D	Precise Location	Point of tying a ponytail, the shikha
E	Tissue Type	sandhi (Joint)
F	Size	Palm size
G	Severity	kālāntaraprāṇahara = fatal after a while
H	Physics/Chemistry	Hypothalamus / Intuition. Instinct. Awareness.
I	Chikitsa recommended	Touch firmly with Index finger tip. May do a slow roll of fingertip.
J	Oil recommended	Brahmi. Brahmi Amla. Almond. Generous pouring of oil.
K	Meditation / Yogasana	Gurudev's Guided Meditation. Sudarshan Kriya.

104. Simanta3 (Vishnurandhra) Features

A	Name	विष्णुरन्ध्र viṣṇurandhra (vishnurandhra)
B	Marma No. No of Points	104. One
C	Body Part	Skull
D	Precise Location	Anterior fontanelle
E	Tissue Type	sandhi (Joint)
F	Size	Palm size
G	Severity	kālāntaraprāṇahara = fatal after a while
H	Physics/Chemistry	Amygdala. Pineal Gland. Master control for entire body mind.
I	Chikitsa recommended	Touch firmly with Index finger tip. May do a slow roll of fingertip.
J	Oil recommended	Brahmi. Brahmi Amla. Almond. Generous pouring of oil.
K	Meditation / Yogasana	Gurudev's Guided Meditation. Sudarshan Kriya.

vishnurandhra, kapala

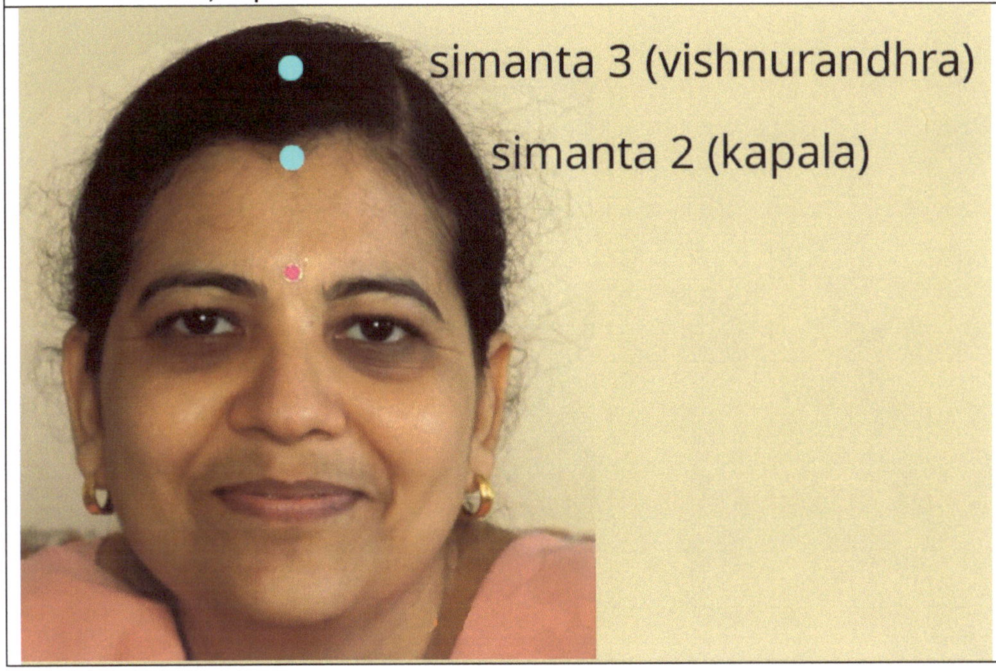

103. Simanta2 (Kapala) Features

A	Name	कपाल kapāla (kapala)
B	Marma No. No of Points	103. One
C	Body Part	Forehead
D	Precise Location	Top of forehead center, just below hairline.
E	Tissue Type	sandhi (Joint)
F	Size	Palm size
G	Severity	kālāntaraprāṇahara = fatal after a while
H	Physics/Chemistry	Reasoning. Thoughts.
I	Chikitsa recommended	Touch firmly with Index finger tip. May do a slow roll of fingertip.
J	Oil recommended	Brahmi. Brahmi Amla. Almond. Balm.
K	Meditation / Yogasana	Kapalabhati Pranayama. Bhastrika Pranayama. Simhasana.

102. Simanta1 (Nasamula) Features

A	Name	नासामूल nāsāmūla (nasamula)
B	Marma No. No of Points	102. One
C	Body Part	Skull
D	Precise Location	Root of Nose, just below Adhipati
E	Tissue Type	sandhi (Joint)
F	Size	Palm size
G	Severity	kālāntaraprāṇahara = fatal after a while
H	Physics/Chemistry	Spiritual. Master control for entire body mind well-being.
I	Chikitsa recommended	Simply ask them to take their attention there.
J	Oil recommended	Noseghee. Anu Taila. Aloe Vera Gel.
K	Meditation / Yogasana	Khechari Mudra. Brahmari Pranayama.

nasamula

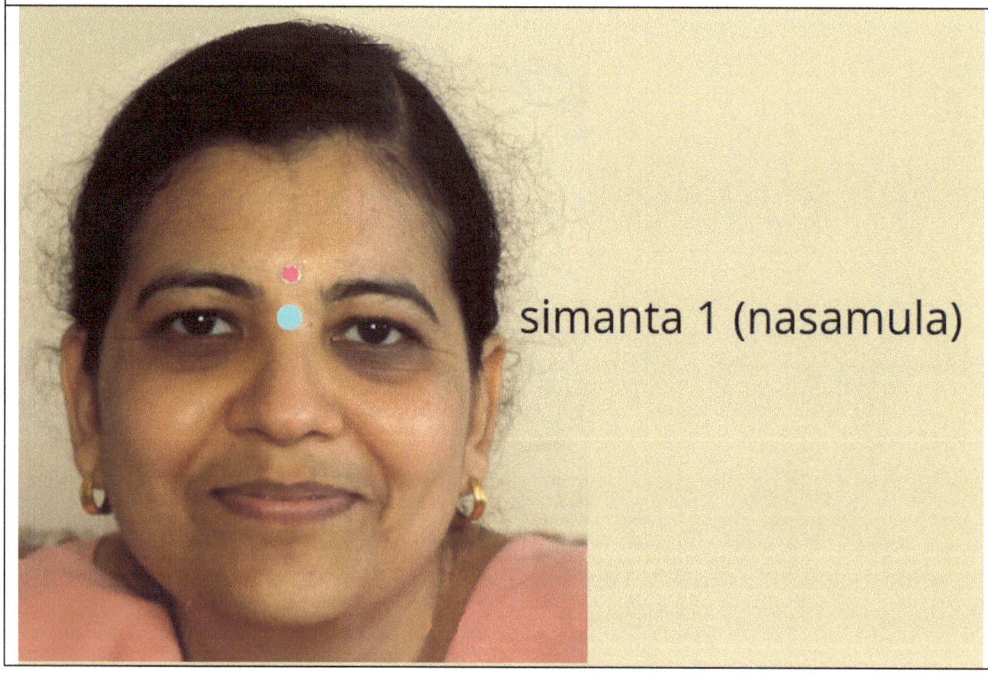

Pair Points in Face = 4+(5x2) = 14

Shringataka	4	4 senses = eyes[4] Kaninaka, ears[3] Karnapali, nose2 Kapola Nasa, tongue[1] oshtha+hanu
Utkshepa	2	Hairline above temple
Avarta	2	midpoint above eye
Shankha	2	temple
Apanga	2	outer corner of eye
Phana	2	nose edge midpoint
Points subTotal	**14**	*(and sthapani accounted for earlier)*

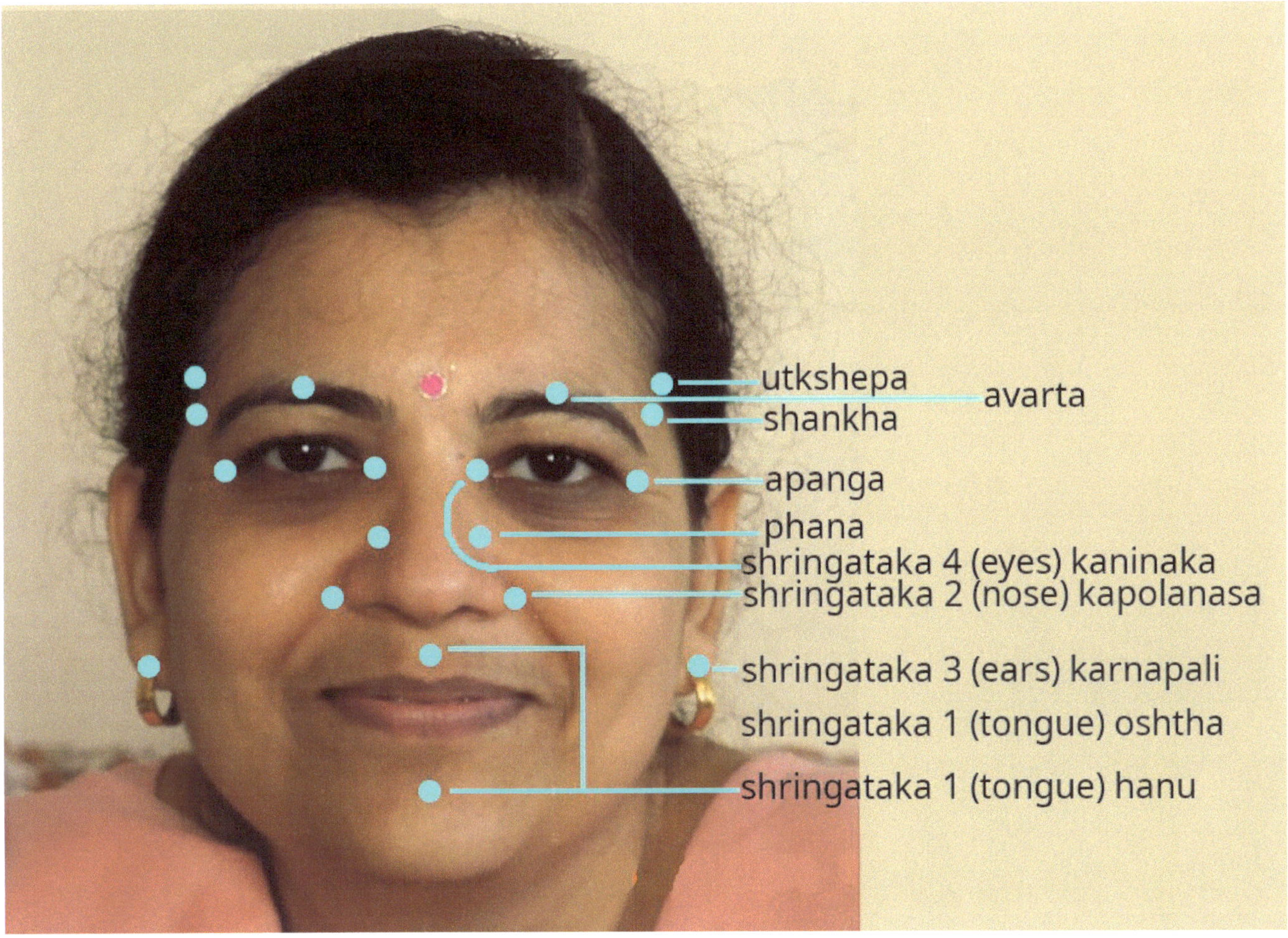

Figure 39: Marma Points in Face (Front View)

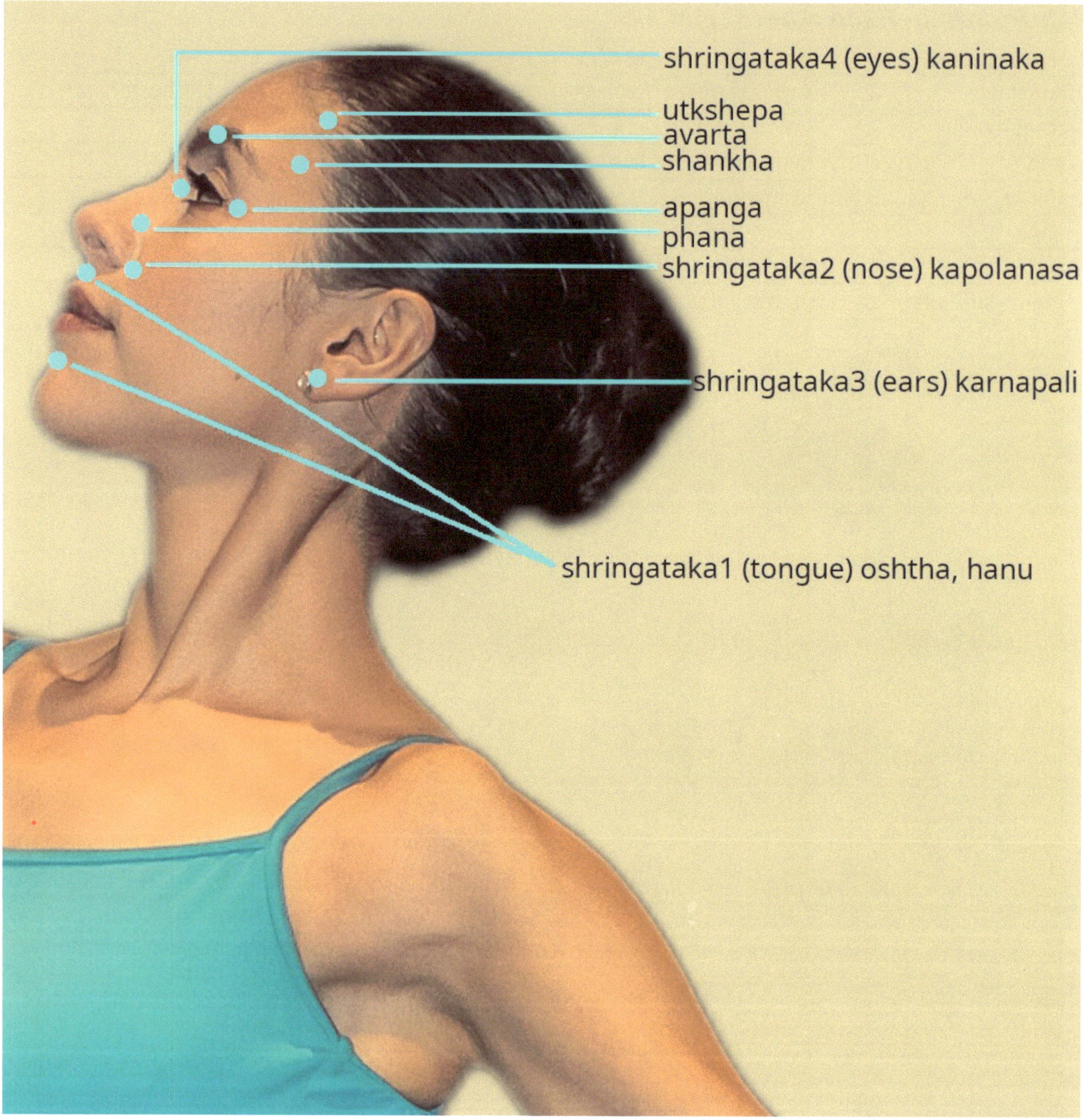

Figure 40: Marma Points in Face (Side View)

101. Shringataka 4a,b (Kaninaka) Features

A	Name	श्रृङ्गाटक कनीनक śṛṅgāṭaka 4a,b kanīnaka (kaninaka)
B	Marma No. No of Points	101. One (pair)
C	Body Part	Eyes
D	Precise Location	Inner eye
E	Tissue Type	sirā (Tube Vein or Artery)
F	Size	Palm size
G	Severity	sadyaḥprāṇahara = instantly fatal
H	Physics/Chemistry	Laughter.
I	Chikitsa recommended	Push gently with Index finger tip.
J	Oil recommended	Rosewater. Aloe Vera Gel.
K	Meditation / Yogasana	Khechari Mudra. Brahmari Pranayama. Palming.

kaninaka, karnapali

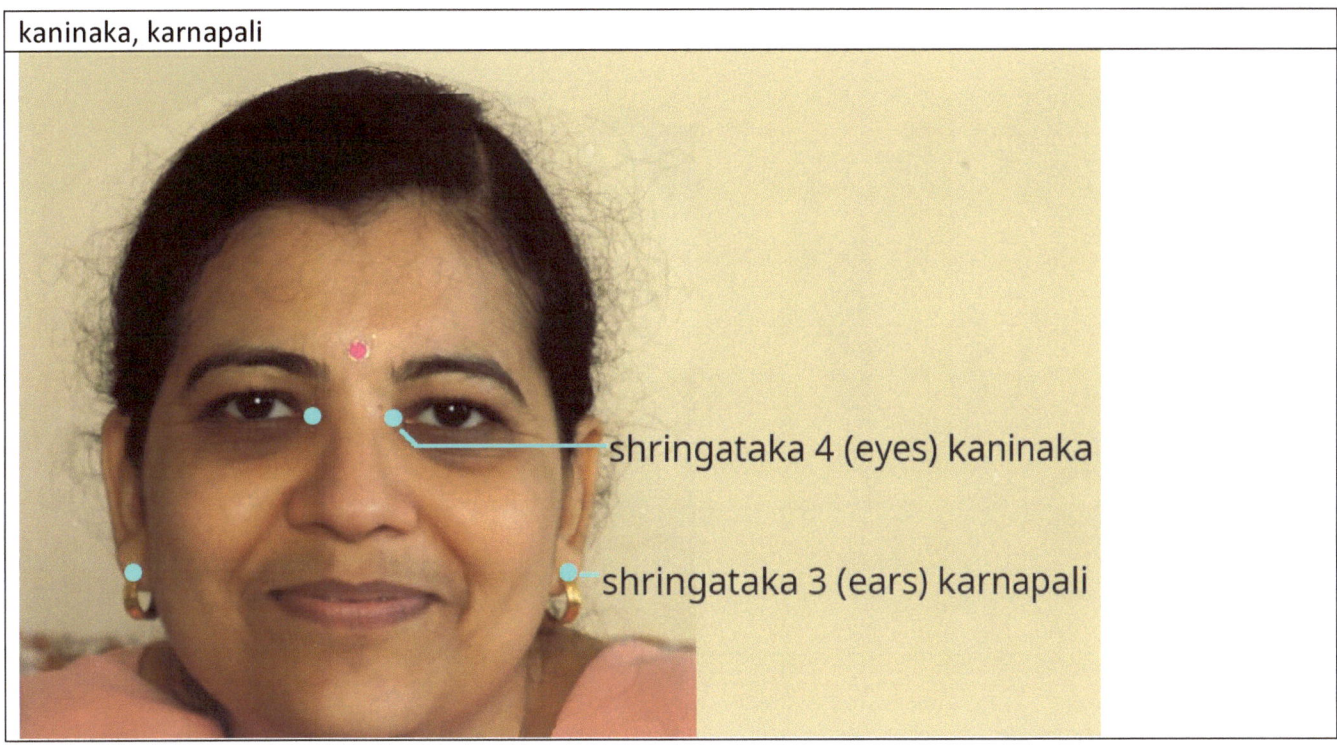

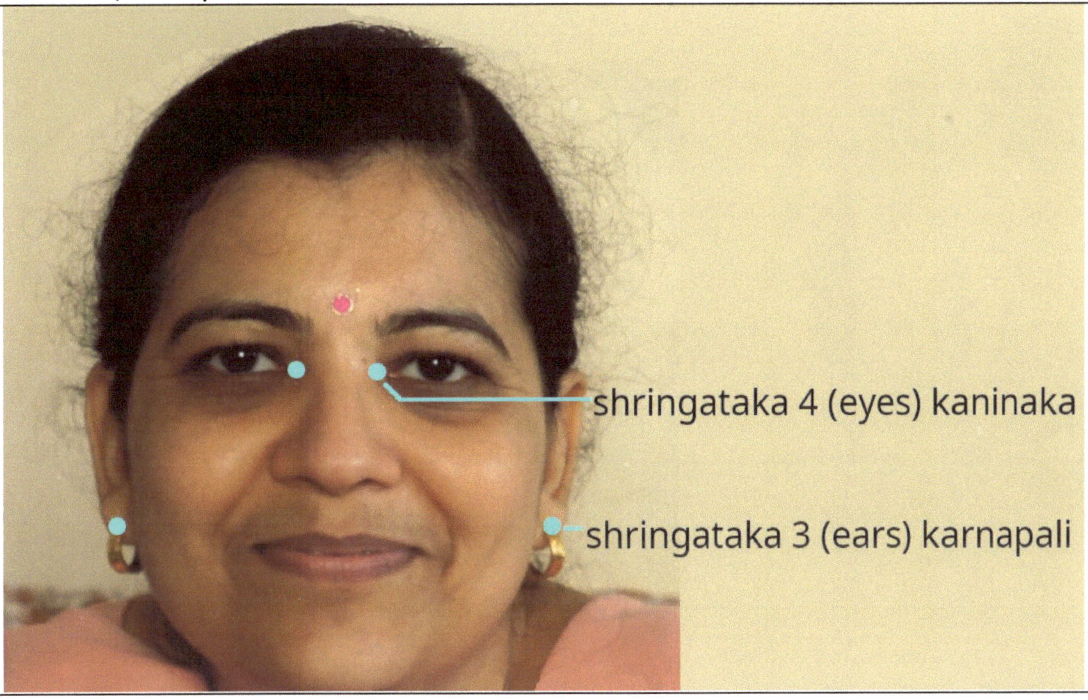

100. Shringataka 3a,b (Karnapali) Features

A	Name	श्रृङ्गाटक कर्णपालि śṛṅgāṭaka 3a,b karṇapāli (karnapali)
B	Marma No. No of Points	100. One (pair)
C	Body Part	Ears
D	Precise Location	earlobe
E	Tissue Type	sirā (Tube Vein or Artery)
F	Size	Palm size
G	Severity	sadyaḥprāṇahara = instantly fatal
H	Physics/Chemistry	Easy going. Carefree.
I	Chikitsa recommended	Pinch and Pull firmly.
J	Oil recommended	Mustard Oil with highly pungent aroma. Balm.
K	Meditation / Yogasana	Khechari Mudra. Brahmari Pranayama.

99. Shringataka 2a,b (Kapolanasa) Features

A	Name	शृङ्गाटक कपोलनासा śṛṅgāṭaka 2a,b kapolanāsā (kapolanasa)
B	Marma No. No of Points	99. One (pair)
C	Body Part	Nose
D	Precise Location	Side of nostril
E	Tissue Type	sirā (Tube Vein or Artery)
F	Size	Palm size
G	Severity	sadyaḥprāṇahara = instantly fatal
H	Physics/Chemistry	Proud.
I	Chikitsa recommended	Touch lightly with Index finger tip.
J	Oil recommended	Noseghee. Anu Taila.
K	Meditation / Yogasana	Khechari Mudra. Brahmari Pranayama.

kapolanasa, oshtha/ hanu

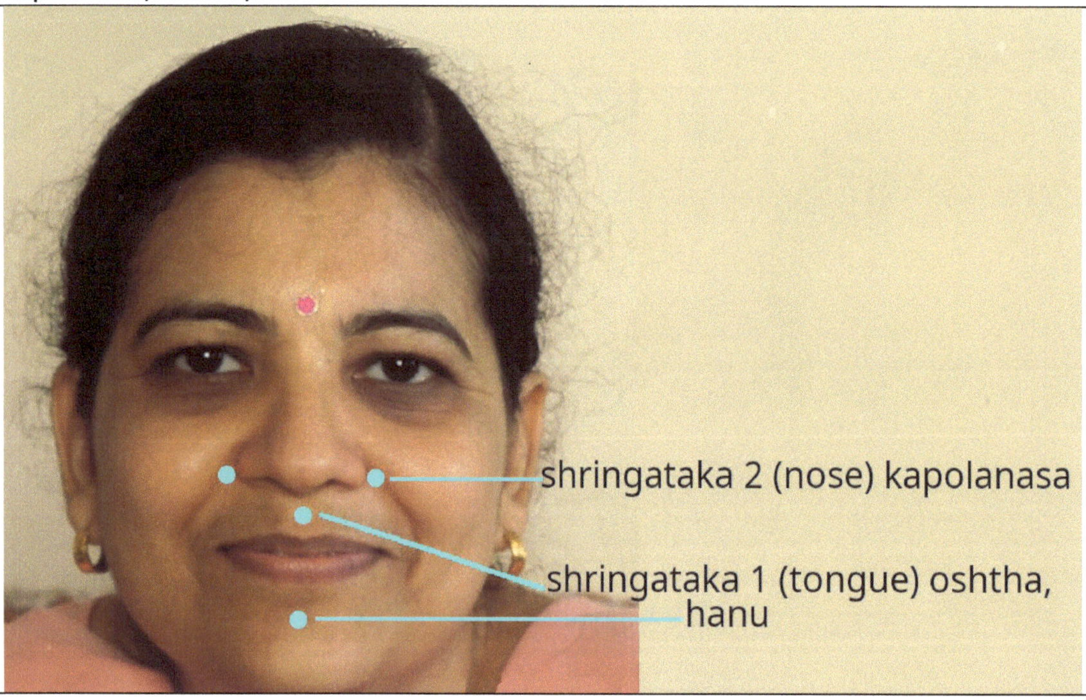

98. Shringataka 1a,b (Oshtha, Hanu) Features

A	Name	शृङ्गाटक ओष्ठ, हनु śṛṅgāṭaka 1a oṣṭha (oshtha), 1b hanu
B	Marma No. No of Points	98. One (pair)
C	Body Part	Face
D	Precise Location	Groove above Upper lip, groove of Chin
E	Tissue Type	sirā (Tube Vein or Artery)
F	Size	Palm size
G	Severity	sadyaḥprāṇahara = instantly fatal
H	Physics/Chemistry	Smiling.
I	Chikitsa recommended	Touch lightly with Index finger tip. May do a slow roll of fingertip.
J	Oil recommended	Rose Oil. Aloe Vera Oil.
K	Meditation / Yogasana	Khechari Mudra. Brahmari Pranayama.

95,96. Utkshepa Features

A	Name	उत्क्षेप utkṣepa (utkshepa)
B	Marma No. No of Points	95,96. Two
C	Body Part	Face
D	Precise Location	At hairline above the Temple
E	Tissue Type	snāyu (Nerve/Tendon)
F	Size	½ angula
G	Severity	viśalyaghna = fatal upon extraction of foreign body lodged here
H	Physics/Chemistry	Thoughtful.
I	Chikitsa recommended	Touch lightly with Index finger tip.
J	Oil recommended	Mustard Oil with highly pungent aroma. Balm.
K	Meditation / Yogasana	Chakra Meditation. Hari Om Meditation. Brahmari Pranayama.

utkshepa, shankha

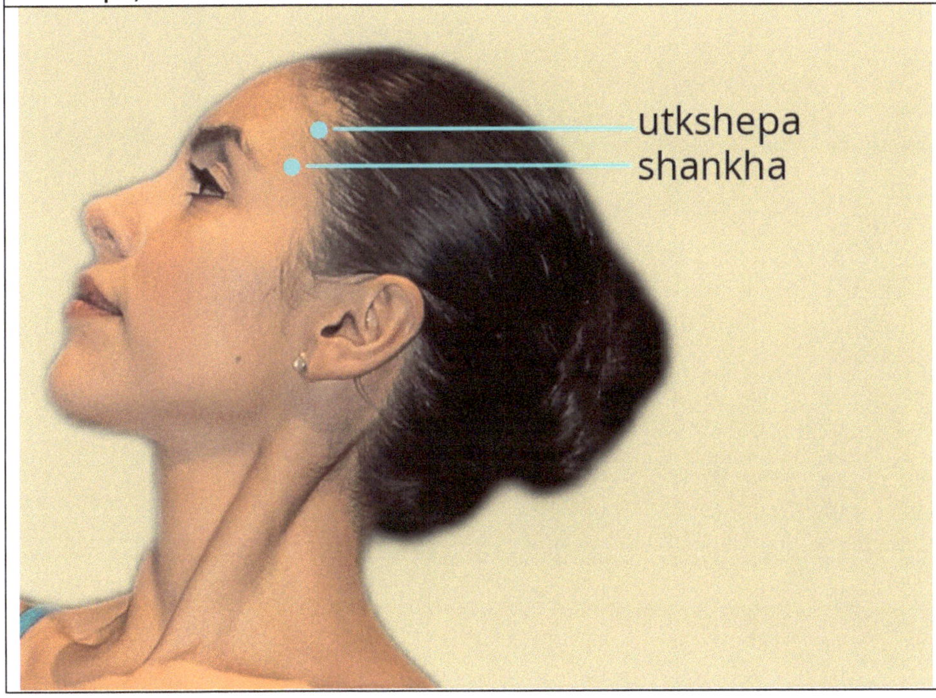

93,94. Shankha Features

A	Name	शङ्ख śaṅkha (shankha)
B	Marma No. No of Points	93,94. Two
C	Body Part	Face
D	Precise Location	Temple
E	Tissue Type	asthi (Bone)
F	Size	½ angula
G	Severity	sadyaḥprāṇahara = instantly fatal
H	Physics/Chemistry	Thoughtful.
I	Chikitsa recommended	Touch lightly with Index finger tip.
J	Oil recommended	Mustard Oil with highly pungent aroma. Balm.
K	Meditation / Yogasana	Chakra Meditation. Hari Om Meditation. Brahmari Pranayama.

91,92. Avarta Features

A	Name	आवर्त āvarta (avarta)
B	Marma No. No of Points	91,92. Two
C	Body Part	Eyes
D	Precise Location	Top eyebrow midpoint
E	Tissue Type	sandhi (Joint)
F	Size	½ angula
G	Severity	vaikalyakara = long term restlessness
H	Physics/Chemistry	Distracted.
I	Chikitsa recommended	Press firmly with Index finger tip.
J	Oil recommended	Rosewater. Aloe Vera Gel.
K	Meditation / Yogasana	Brahmari Pranayama. Eyes Rotation, Blinking, Squeezing. Palming.

avarta, apanga

89,90. Apanga Features

A	Name	अपाङ्ग apāṅga (apanga)
B	Marma No. No of Points	89,90. Two
C	Body Part	Eyes
D	Precise Location	Outer corner of eye
E	Tissue Type	sirā (Tube Vein or Artery)
F	Size	½ angula
G	Severity	vaikalyakara = long term restlessness
H	Physics/Chemistry	Wonder.
I	Chikitsa recommended	Press firmly with Index finger tip.
J	Oil recommended	Rosewater.
K	Meditation / Yogasana	Brahmari Pranayama. Eyes Rotation, Blinking, Squeezing. Palming.

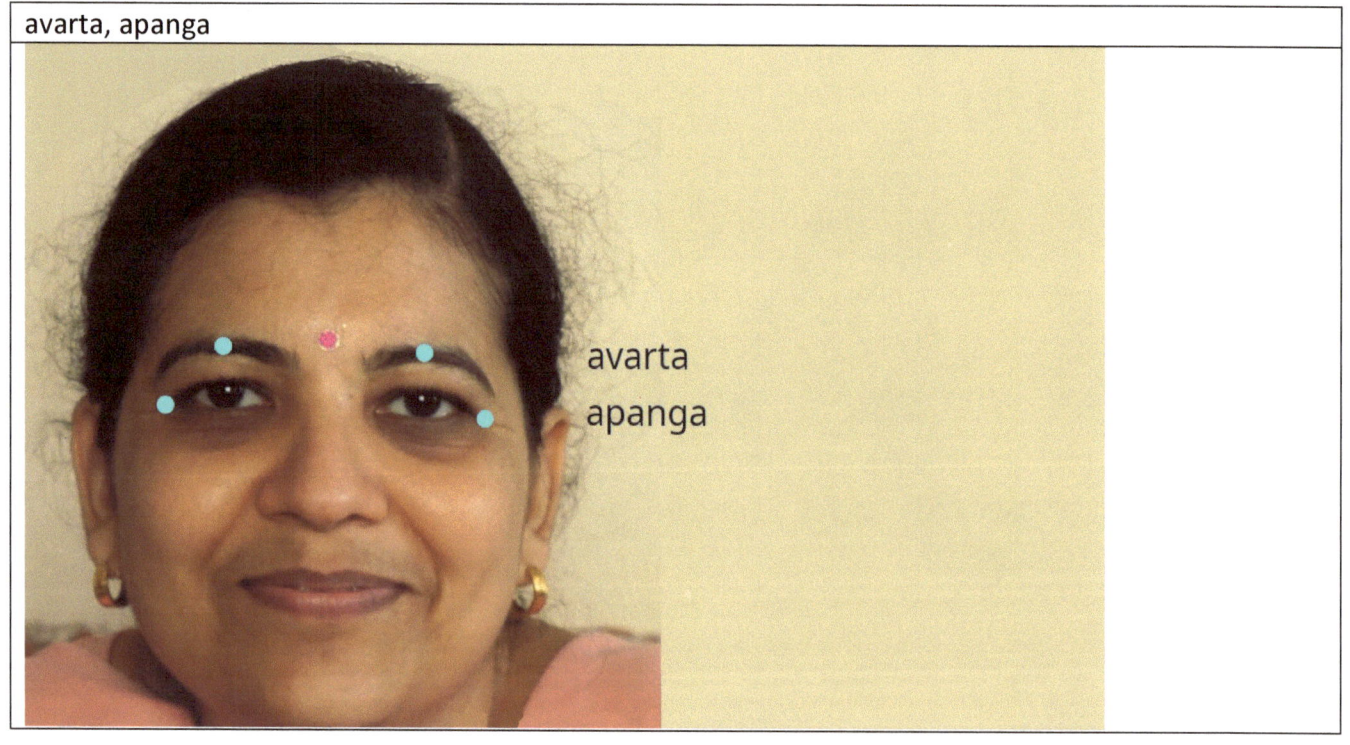

87,88. Phana Features

A	Name	फण phaṇa (phana)
B	Marma No. No of Points	87,88. 1
C	Body Part	Face
D	Precise Location	sinus at midpoint of edge of nose
E	Tissue Type	sirā (Tube Vein or Artery)
F	Size	½ angula
G	Severity	vaikalyakara = long term restlessness
H	Physics/Chemistry	Thoughtful.
I	Chikitsa recommended	Touch lightly with Index finger tip.
J	Oil recommended	Mustard Oil with highly pungent aroma. Balm.
K	Meditation / Yogasana	Khechari Pranayama. Brahmari Pranayama.

phana

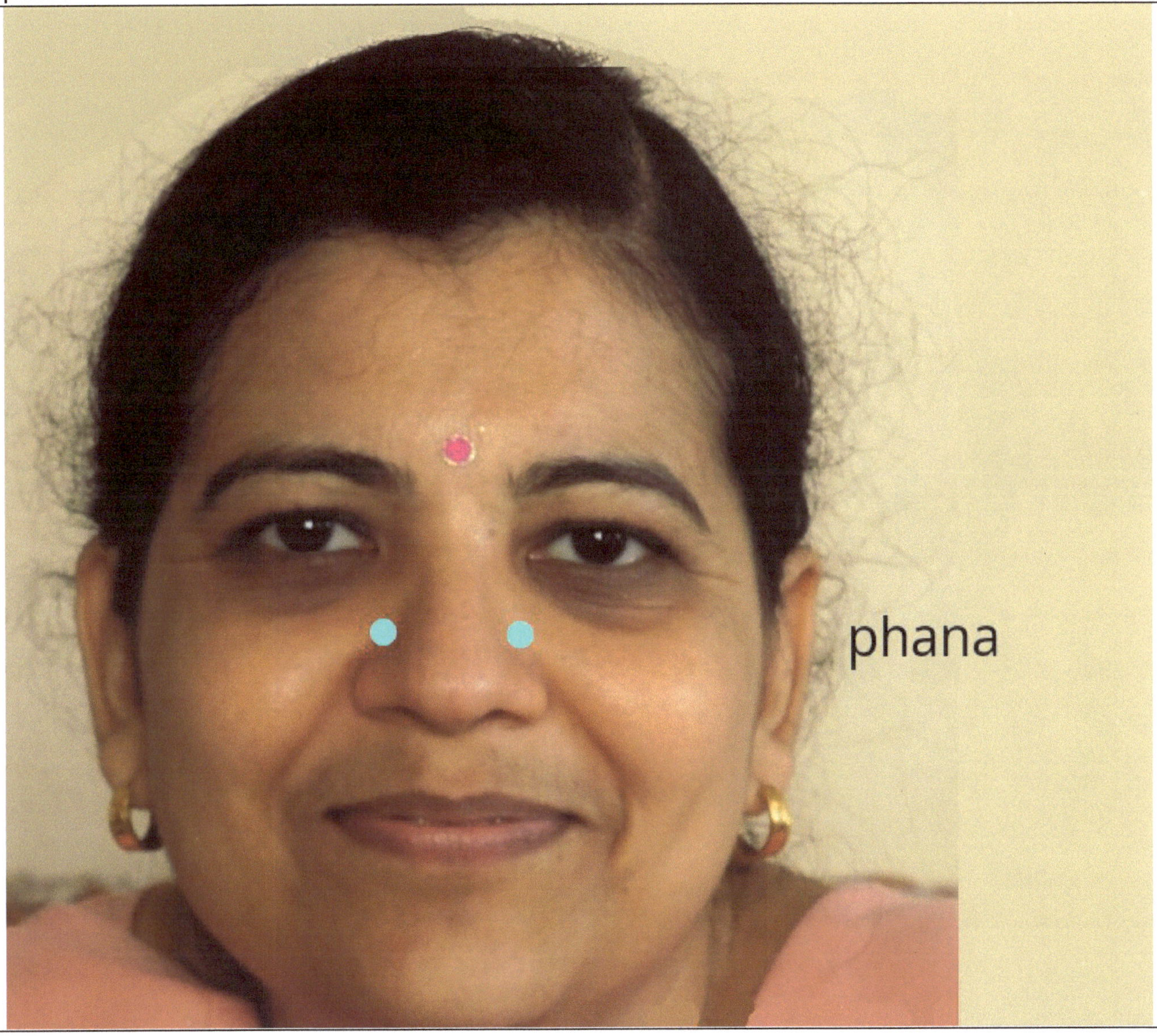

Pair Points in Neck = 8x2 -1 = 15

Vidhura	2	Below ear at back
Krikatika	2	neck joint at back
Dhamani Manya	2	upper neck on sternocleidomastoid muscle
Dhamani Nila	2	lower neck on sternocleidomastoid muscle
Matrika / Sira Matrika	4 pairs - 1 = 8 – 1 = 7	Front Side of Body Matrika 1st pair = Akshaka Matrika 2nd pair = Kantha *(and Kanthanadi accounted for earlier)*
		Rear Side of Body Matrika 3rd pair = Prishtagriva Matrika 4th pair = Griva and Manyamani
Points subTotal	**15**	

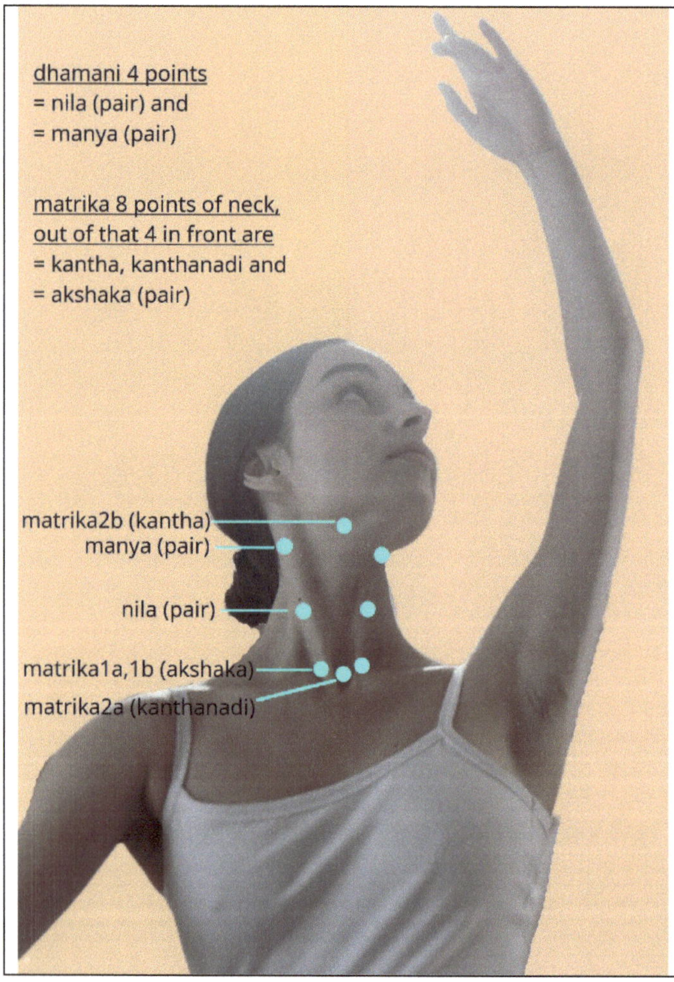

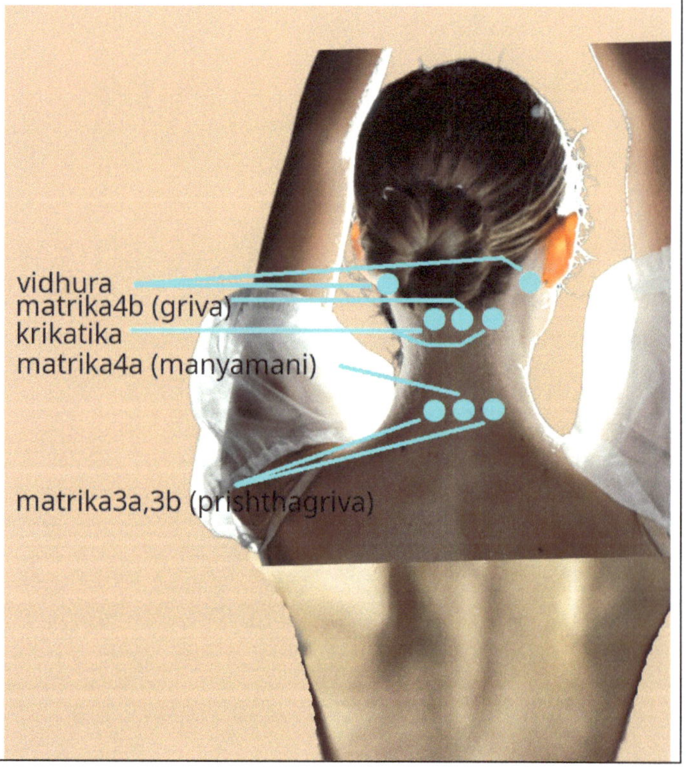

Figure 41: Marma Points in Neck (Front View)

85,86. Vidhura Features

A	Name	विधुर vidhura
B	Marma No. No of Points	85,86. Two
C	Body Part	Neck behind ear
D	Precise Location	2 angula behind earlobe.
E	Tissue Type	snāyu (Nerve/Tendon)
F	Size	½ angula.
G	Severity	vaikalyakara = long term restlessness
H	Physics/Chemistry	Hope. Faith.
I	Chikitsa recommended	Touch lightly with Index finger tip. May do a slow roll of fingertip.
J	Oil recommended	Ashwagandha. Mahanarayana. Brahmi.
K	Meditation / Yogasana	Chakra Meditation. Hari Om Meditation.

vidhura, krikatika

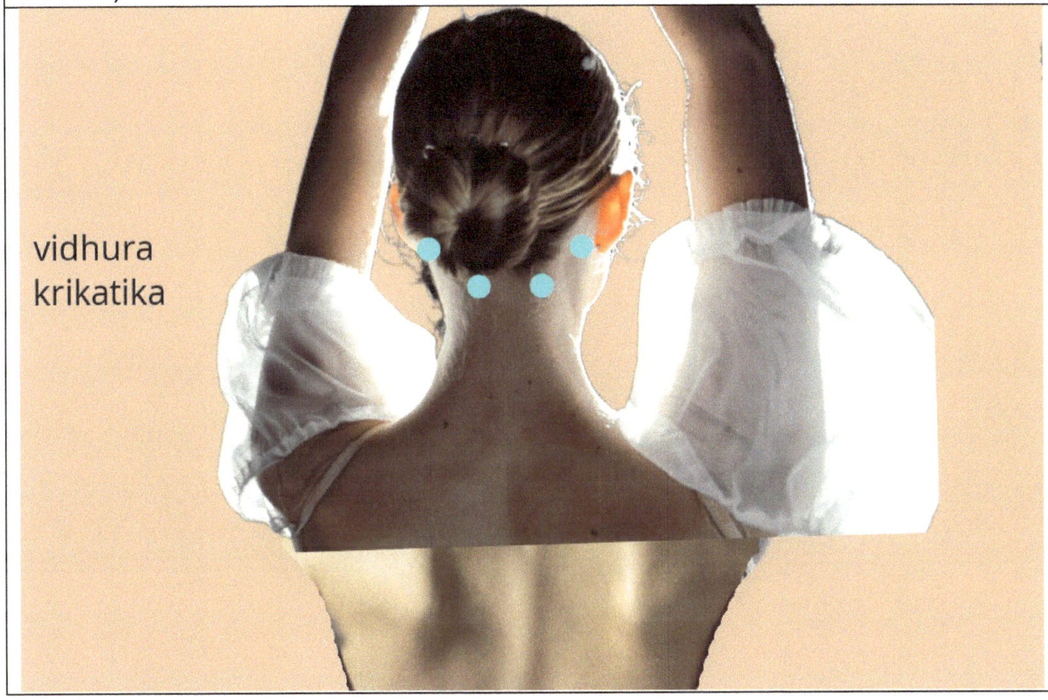

83,84. Krikatika Features

A	Name	कृकाटिका kṛkāṭikā (krikatika)
B	Marma No. No of Points	83,84. Two
C	Body Part	Neck
D	Precise Location	Junction of neck with head at rear.
E	Tissue Type	sandhi (Joint)
F	Size	½ angula.
G	Severity	vaikalyakara = long term restlessness
H	Physics/Chemistry	Needing external support.
I	Chikitsa recommended	Touch lightly with Index finger tip. May do a slow roll of fingertip.
J	Oil recommended	Ashwagandha. Kshirabala.
K	Meditation / Yogasana	Bhramari Pranayama. Neck Roll.

81,82. Matrika 4a,4b (manyāmaṇi, grīvā) Features

A	Name	मन्यामणि manyāmaṇi (manyamani), ग्रीवा grīvā (griva)
B	Marma No. No of Points	81,82. Two
C	Body Part	Neck rear
D	Precise Location	Below ear at back
E	Tissue Type	sirā (Tube Vein or Artery)
F	Size	Palm size
G	Severity	sadyaḥprāṇahara = instantly fatal
H	Physics/Chemistry	Unyielding.
I	Chikitsa recommended	Touch lightly with Index finger tip.
J	Oil recommended	Ashwagandha. Kshirabala.
K	Meditation / Yogasana	Bhramari Pranayama. Neck Roll. Extended Palms. Mountain Pose.

manyamani, griva, prishtagriva pair

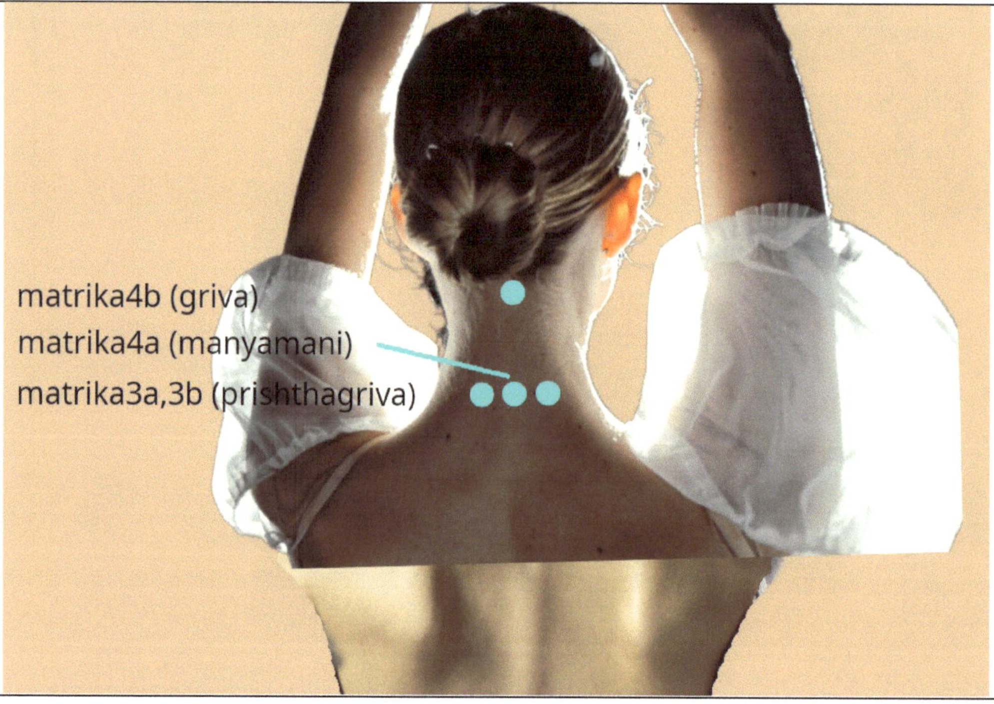

79,80. Matrika 3a,3b (pṛṣṭhagrīva) Features

A	Name	पृष्ठग्रीव pṛṣṭhagrīva (prishtagriva)
B	Marma No. No of Points	79,80. Two
C	Body Part	Neck rear
D	Precise Location	Joint of neck with head
E	Tissue Type	sirā (Tube Vein or Artery)
F	Size	Palm size
G	Severity	sadyaḥprāṇahara = instantly fatal
H	Physics/Chemistry	Stubborn.
I	Chikitsa recommended	Touch firmly with Index finger tip.
J	Oil recommended	Ashwagandha. Kshirabala. Firm Massage
K	Meditation / Yogasana	Bhramari Pranayama. Neck Roll. Extended Palms. Mountain Pose

78. Matrika 2b (kaṇṭha) Features

A	Name	कण्ठ kaṇṭha (kantha)
B	Marma No. No of Points	78. One
C	Body Part	Throat
D	Precise Location	Joint of throat with head
E	Tissue Type	sirā (Tube Vein or Artery)
F	Size	Palm size
G	Severity	sadyaḥprāṇahara = instantly fatal
H	Physics/Chemistry	Grateful.
I	Chikitsa recommended	Touch gently with Index finger tip.
J	Oil recommended	A2 Ghee.
K	Meditation / Yogasana	Ujjayi Pranayama. Simhasana. Hari Om Meditation. Sudarshan Kriya.

manyamani, griva, prishtagriva pair

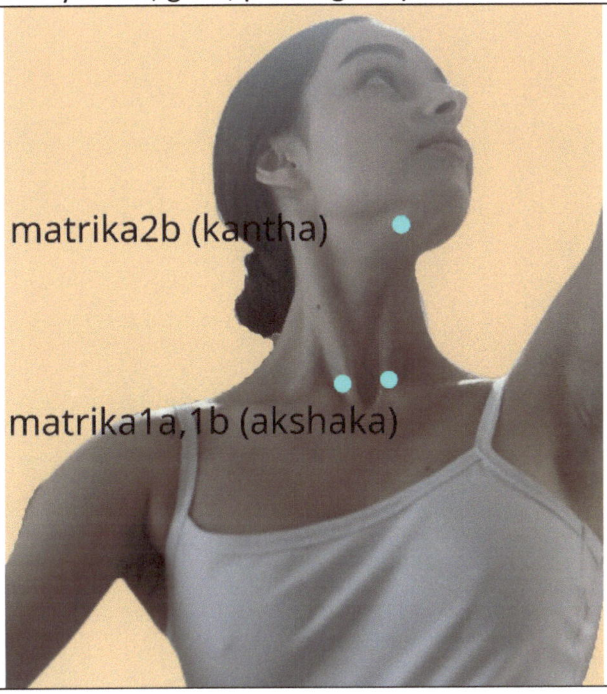

75,76. Matrika 1a,1b (Akshaka) Features

A	Name	अक्षक akshaka
B	Marma No. No of Points	75,76. Two
C	Body Part	Throat
D	Precise Location	Lowermost part of sternocleidomastoid muscle (3/3rd distance)
E	Tissue Type	sirā (Tube Vein or Artery)
F	Size	Palm size
G	Severity	sadyaḥprāṇahara = instantly fatal
H	Physics/Chemistry	Grateful.
I	Chikitsa recommended	Touch gently with Index finger tip.
J	Oil recommended	A2 Ghee.
K	Meditation / Yogasana	Ujjayi Pranayama. Simhasana. Hari Om Meditation. Sudarshan Kriya.

73,74. Dhamani Manya Features

A	Name	मन्या manyā (manya)
B	Marma No. No of Points	73,74. Two
C	Body Part	Throat
D	Precise Location	upper neck on sternocleidomastoid muscle (1/3rd distance)
E	Tissue Type	sirā (Tube Vein or Artery)
F	Size	Palm size
G	Severity	sadyaḥprāṇahara = instantly fatal
H	Physics/Chemistry	Grateful.
I	Chikitsa recommended	Touch lightly with Index finger tip.
J	Oil recommended	A2 Ghee.
K	Meditation / Yogasana	Ujjayi Pranayama. Simhasana. Sarvangasana.

manya, nila

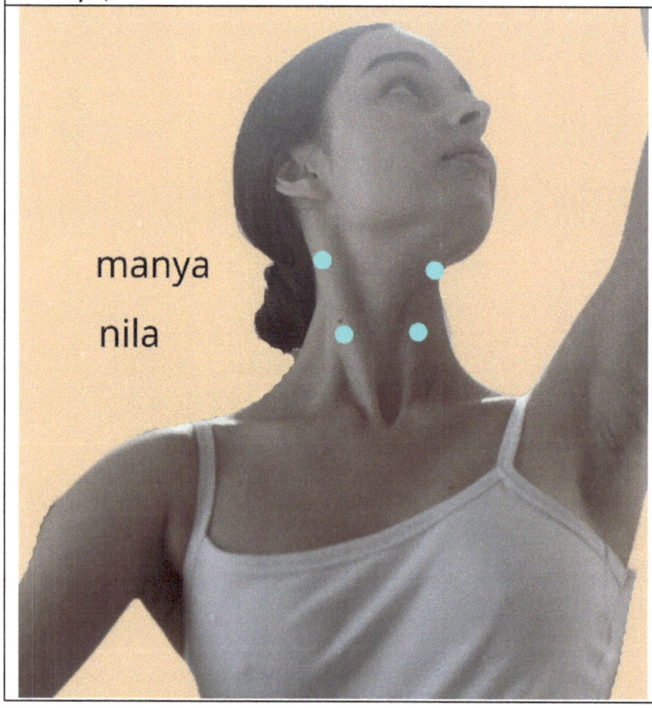

71,72. Dhamani Nila Features

A	Name	नीला nīlā (nila)
B	Marma No. No of Points	71,72. Two
C	Body Part	Throat
D	Precise Location	lower neck on sternocleidomastoid muscle (2/3rd distance)
E	Tissue Type	sirā (Tube Vein or Artery)
F	Size	Palm size
G	Severity	sadyaḥprāṇahara = instantly fatal
H	Physics/Chemistry	Grateful.
I	Chikitsa recommended	Touch lightly with Index finger tip.
J	Oil recommended	A2 Ghee.
K	Meditation	Ujjayi Pranayama. Simhasana. Sarvangasana. Hari Om Meditation.

Pair Points in Back = 7x2 = 14

Amsa	2	Portion of shoulder right on top
Amsaphalaka	2	Extension of shoulder at back
Brihati	2	major middle Back area
Parshvasandhi	2	side Joints at back
Nitamba	2	Hip
Kukundara	2	shape curve at edge of back
Katikataruna	2	veins very close to lowermost spine
Points subTotal	**14**	

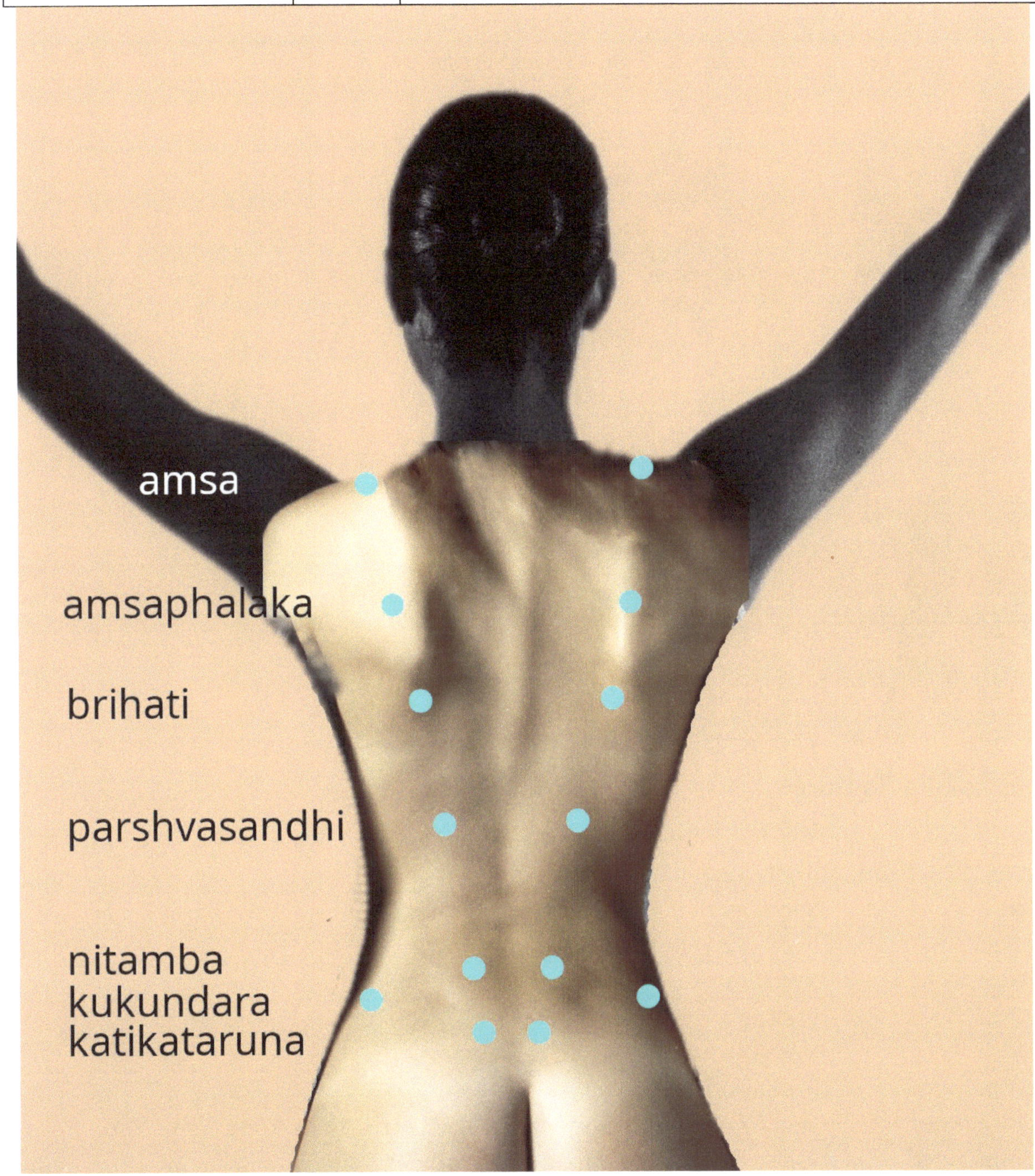

Figure 42: Marma Points in Back

69,70. Amsa Features

A	Name	अंस aṃsa (amsa)
B	Marma No. No of Points	69,70. Two
C	Body Part	top of Shoulder
D	Precise Location	top shoulder groove
E	Tissue Type	snāyu (Nerve/Tendon)
F	Size	½ angula
G	Severity	vaikalyakara = long term restlessness
H	Physics/Chemistry	Responsible.
I	Chikitsa recommended	Touch firmly with Index finger tip. May do a slow roll of fingertip.
J	Oil recommended	Ashwagandha. Mahanarayana. Firm Massage.
K	Meditation / Yogasana	Shoulder roll, Swimming, Extended Palms

amsa, amsaphalaka

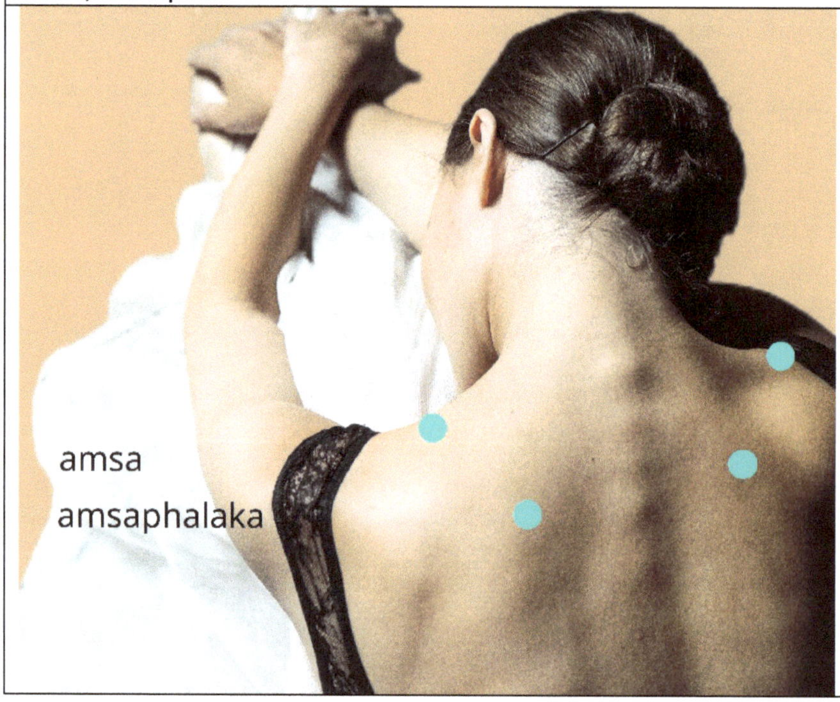

67,68. Amsaphalaka Features

A	Name	अंसफलक aṃsaphalaka (amsaphalaka)
B	Marma No. No of Points	67,68. Two
C	Body Part	Shoulder blade
D	Precise Location	Middle of shoulder blade
E	Tissue Type	asthi (Bone)
F	Size	½ angula
G	Severity	vaikalyakara = long term restlessness
H	Physics/Chemistry	Expansion.
I	Chikitsa recommended	Touch firmly with Index finger tip. May do a slow roll of fingertip.
J	Oil recommended	Ashwagandha. Mahanarayana. Firm Massage.
K	Meditation / Yogasana	Shoulder roll, Swimming, Extended Palms

65,66. Brihati Features

A	Name	बृहती bṛhatī (brihati)
B	Marma No. No of Points	65.66. Two
C	Body Part	Middle back
D	Precise Location	Below shoulder blades
E	Tissue Type	sirā (Tube Vein or Artery)
F	Size	½ angula
G	Severity	kālāntaraprāṇahara = fatal after a while
H	Physics/Chemistry	Storing personal and private memories.
I	Chikitsa recommended	Touch firmly with Index finger tip. May do a slow roll of fingertip.
J	Oil recommended	Ashwagandha. Kshirabala. Firm Massage.
K	Meditation / Yogasana	Bhujangasana. Paschimottanasana. Bench Press.

brihati, parshvasandhi

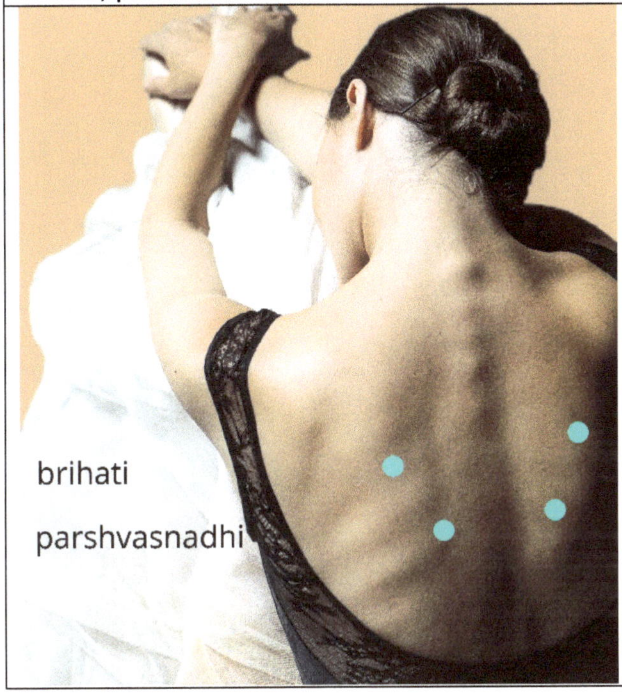

63,64. Parshvasandhi Features

A	Name	पार्श्वसन्धि pārśvasandhi (parshvasandhi)
B	Marma No. No of Points	63,64. Two
C	Body Part	Middle back
D	Precise Location	Flanks of lumbar spine
E	Tissue Type	sirā (Tube Vein or Artery)
F	Size	½ angula
G	Severity	kālāntaraprāṇahara = fatal after a while
H	Physics/Chemistry	Storing personal and private memories.
I	Chikitsa recommended	Touch firmly with Index finger tip. May do a slow roll of fingertip.
J	Oil recommended	Ashwagandha. Mahanarayana. Firm Massage.
K	Meditation / Yogasana	Bhujangasana. Paschimottanasana. Bench Press.

61,62. Nitamba Features

A	Name	नितम्ब nitamba
B	Marma No. No of Points	61,62. Two
C	Body Part	Lower back
D	Precise Location	hip
E	Tissue Type	asthi (Bone)
F	Size	½ angula
G	Severity	kālāntaraprāṇahara = fatal after a while
H	Physics/Chemistry	Firm. Steady.
I	Chikitsa recommended	Touch firmly with Index finger tip. May do a slow roll of fingertip.
J	Oil recommended	Ashwagandha. Mahanarayana. Firm Massage.
K	Meditation / Yogasana	Bhujangasana. Paschimottanasana. Chakra Meditation. Waist Roll.

nitamba, kukundara

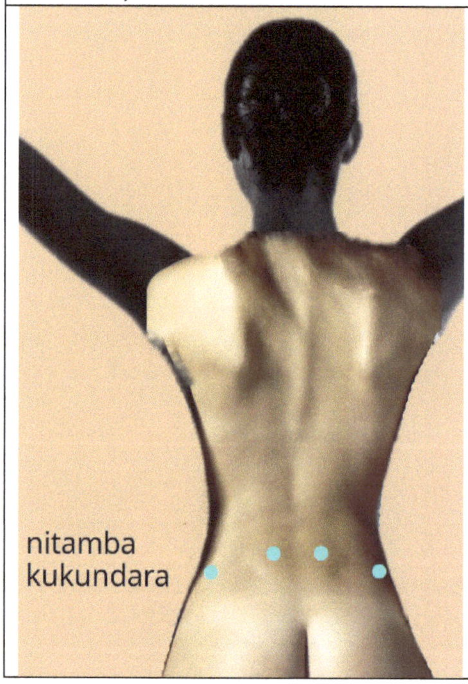

59,60. Kukundara Features

A	Name	कुकुन्दर kukundara
B	Marma No. No of Points	59,60. Two
C	Body Part	Lower back
D	Precise Location	Flank of lower back
E	Tissue Type	Sandhi (Joint)
F	Size	½ angula
G	Severity	kālāntaraprāṇahara = fatal after a while
H	Physics/Chemistry	Bold. Social.
I	Chikitsa recommended	Touch firmly with Index finger tip. May do a slow roll of fingertip.
J	Oil recommended	Ashwagandha. Mahanarayana. Firm Massage.
K	Meditation / Yogasana	Bhujangasana. Paschimottanasana. Waist Rotation.

57,58. Katikataruna Features

A	Name	कटीकतरुण kaṭīkataruṇa (katikataruna)
B	Marma No. No of Points	57,58. Two
C	Body Part	Lower back
D	Precise Location	Lower spine
E	Tissue Type	asthi (Bone)
F	Size	½ angula
G	Severity	kālāntaraprāṇahara = fatal after a while
H	Physics/Chemistry	Small. Fragile. Timid.
I	Chikitsa recommended	Touch firmly with Index finger tip. May do a slow roll of fingertip.
J	Oil recommended	Ashwagandha. Mahanarayana. Firm Massage.
K	Meditation / Yogasana	Bhujangasana. Paschimottanasana. Waist Rotation.

katikataruna

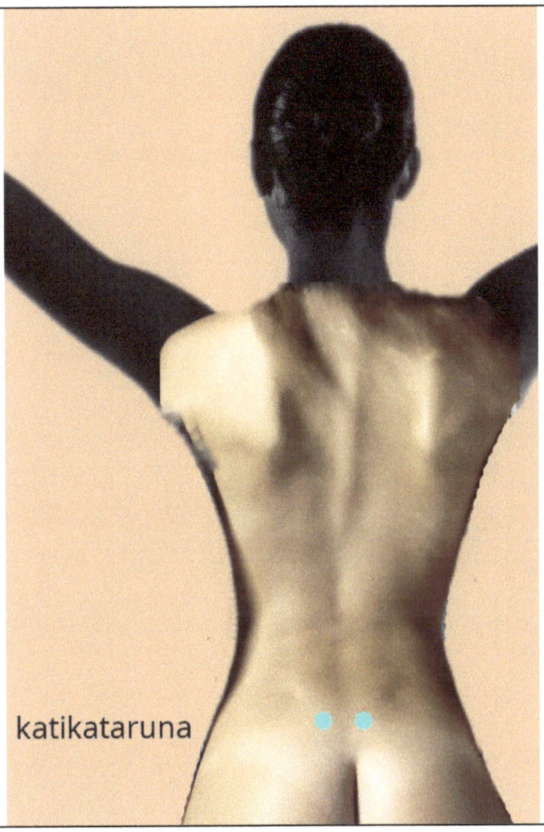

Pair Points in Chest = 4x2 = 8

Apastambha	2	just below the clavicle
Apalapa	2	cleavage line
Stanarohita	2	2 angula above nipple
Stanamula	2	2 angula below nipple
Points subTotal	**8**	
Marma Points in Body Midline are accounted for earlier		

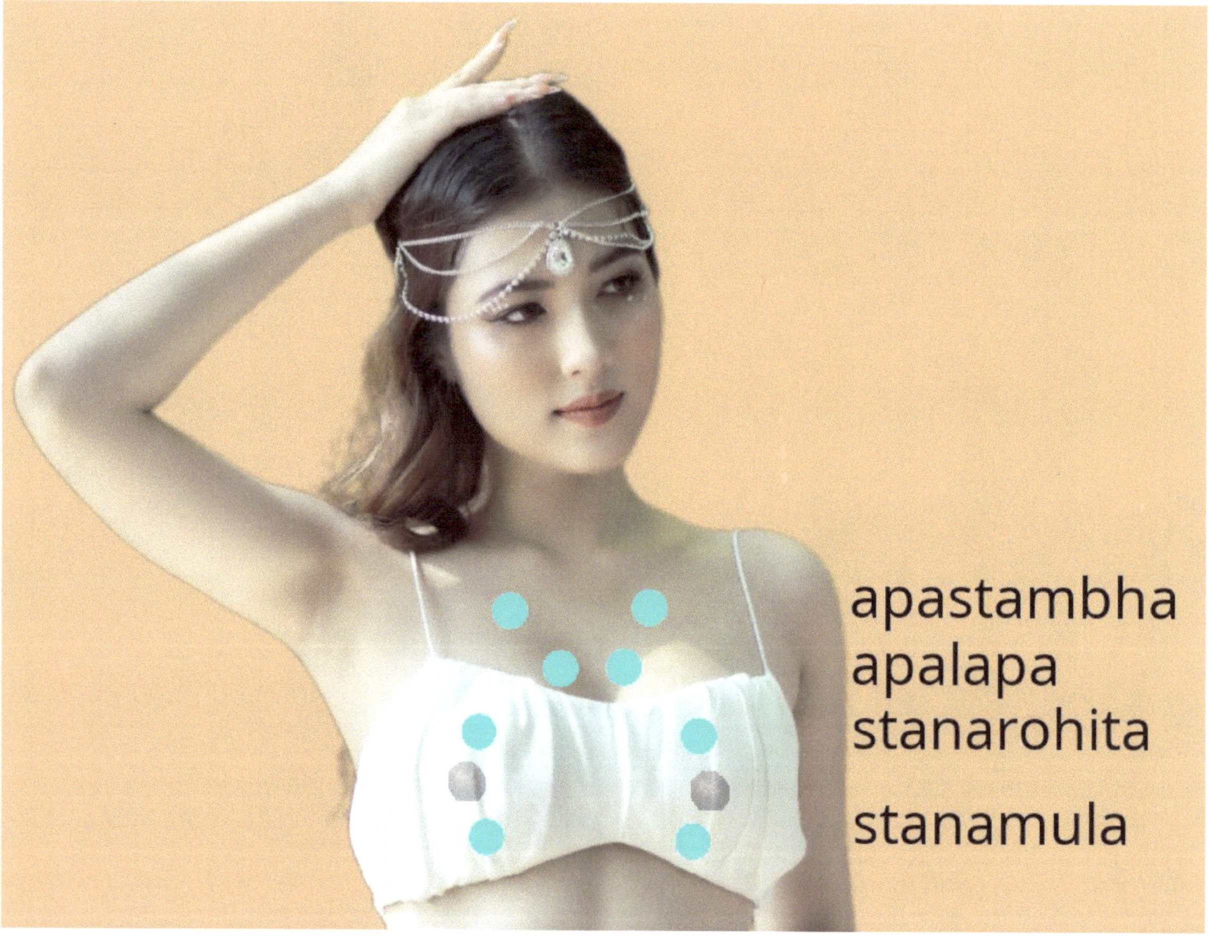

Figure 43: Marma Points in Chest except those already accounted for

55,56. Apastambha Features

A	Name	अपस्तम्भ apastambha
B	Marma No. No of Points	55,56. Two
C	Body Part	Just below the clavicle
D	Precise Location	Veins feeding the chest
E	Tissue Type	सिरा sirā (Tube vein or artery)
F	Size	अर्ध-अङ्गुल ½ angula.
G	Severity	kālāntaraprāṇahara = fatal after a while
H	Physics/Chemistry	Expansion. Sharing.
I	Chikitsa recommended	Touch lightly with Index finger tip. May do a slow roll of fingertip.
J	Oil recommended	A2 Ghee. Kshirabala.
K	Meditation / Yogasana	Ujjayi Pranayama. Bhujangasana. Dhanurasana.

apastambha, apalapa

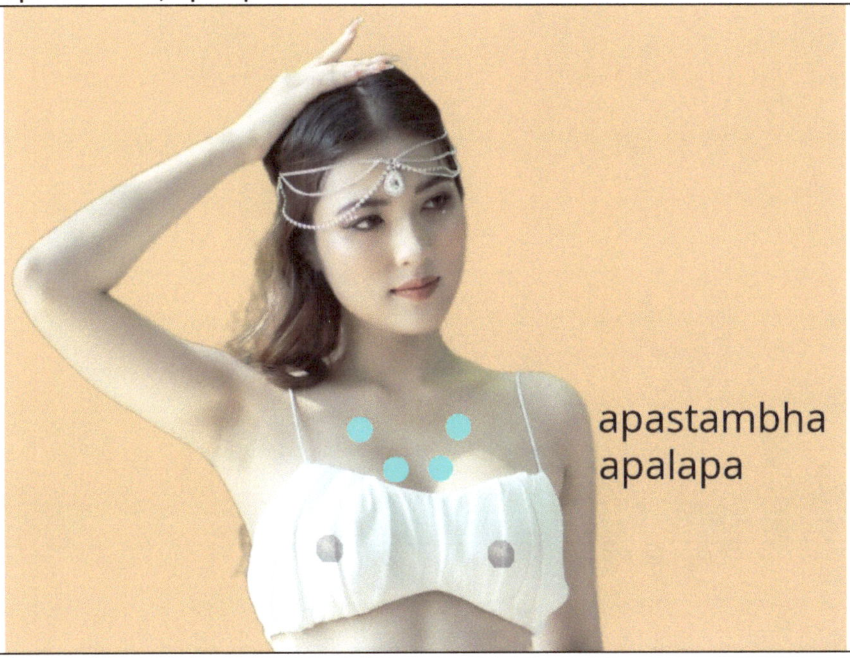

53,54. Apalapa Features

A	Name	अपलाप apalāpa (apalapa)
B	Marma No. No of Points	53,54. Two
C	Body Part	Cleavage
D	Precise Location	on the breast cleavage upper portion
E	Tissue Type	सिरा sirā (Tube vein or artery)
F	Size	अर्ध-अङ्गुल ½ angula.
G	Severity	kālāntaraprāṇaharāṇi = fatal after a while
H	Physics/Chemistry	Storing personal and private memories.
I	Chikitsa recommended	Touch lightly with Index finger tip. May do a slow roll of fingertip.
J	Oil recommended	A2 Ghee. Kshirabala.
K	Meditation / Yogasana	Ujjayi Pranayama. Bhujangasana. Dhanurasana.

51,52. Stanarohita Features

A	Name	स्तनरोहित stanarohita
B	Marma No. No of Points	51,52. Two
C	Body Part	Breast
D	Precise Location	2 angula above nipple
E	Tissue Type	मांस māṃsa (Muscle)
F	Size	अर्ध-अङ्गुल ½ angula.
G	Severity	kālāntaraprāṇahara = fatal after a while
H	Physics/Chemistry	Emotional. Master Control of Delicate Emotions.
I	Chikitsa recommended	Touch lightly with Index finger tip. May do a slow roll of fingertip.
J	Oil recommended	A2 Ghee. Fresh Cream.
K	Meditation / Yogasana	Ujjayi Pranayama. Bhujangasana. Sudarshan Kriya.

stanarohita, stanamula

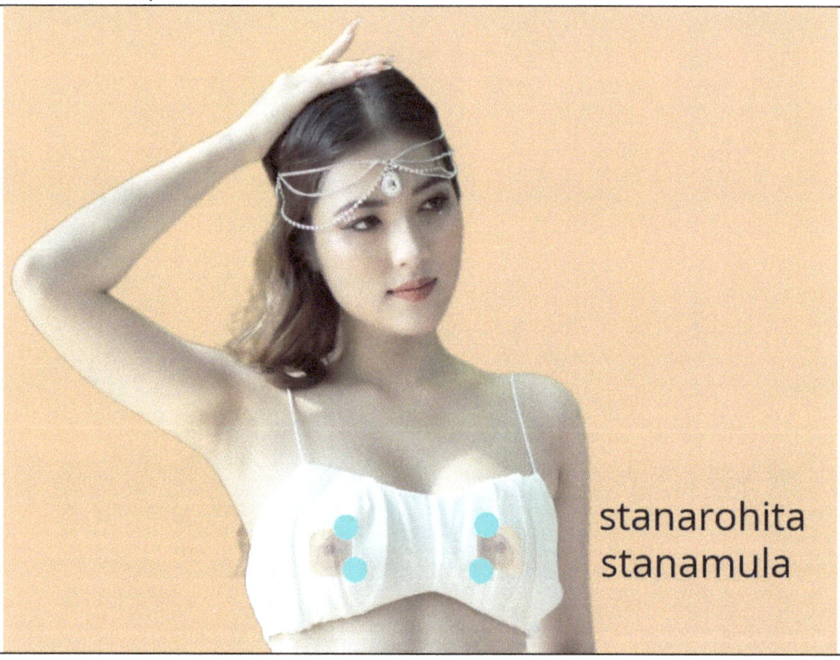

49,50. Stanamula Features

A	Name	स्तनमूल stanamūla (stanamula)
B	Marma No. No of Points	49,50. Two
C	Body Part	Breast
D	Precise Location	2 angula below nipple
E	Tissue Type	सिरा sirā (Tube vein or artery)
F	Size	अर्ध-अङ्गुल ½ angula.
G	Severity	kālāntaraprāṇahara = fatal after a while
H	Physics/Chemistry	Emotional. Master Control of Delicate Emotions.
I	Chikitsa recommended	Touch lightly with Index finger tip. May do a slow roll of fingertip.
J	Oil recommended	A2 Ghee. Fresh Cream.
K	Meditation / Yogasana	Ujjayi Pranayama. Bhujangasana. Sudarshan Kriya.

Pair Points in Arms = 7x2 = 14

Kakshadhara	2	shoulder joint top
Lohitaksha arm	2	lower front end of shoulder joint
Urvi arm	2	armpit
Ani arm	2	lower part of upper arm
Kurpara	2	elbow joint
Indrabasti arm	2	forearm center
Manibandha	2	wrist
Points subTotal	**14**	

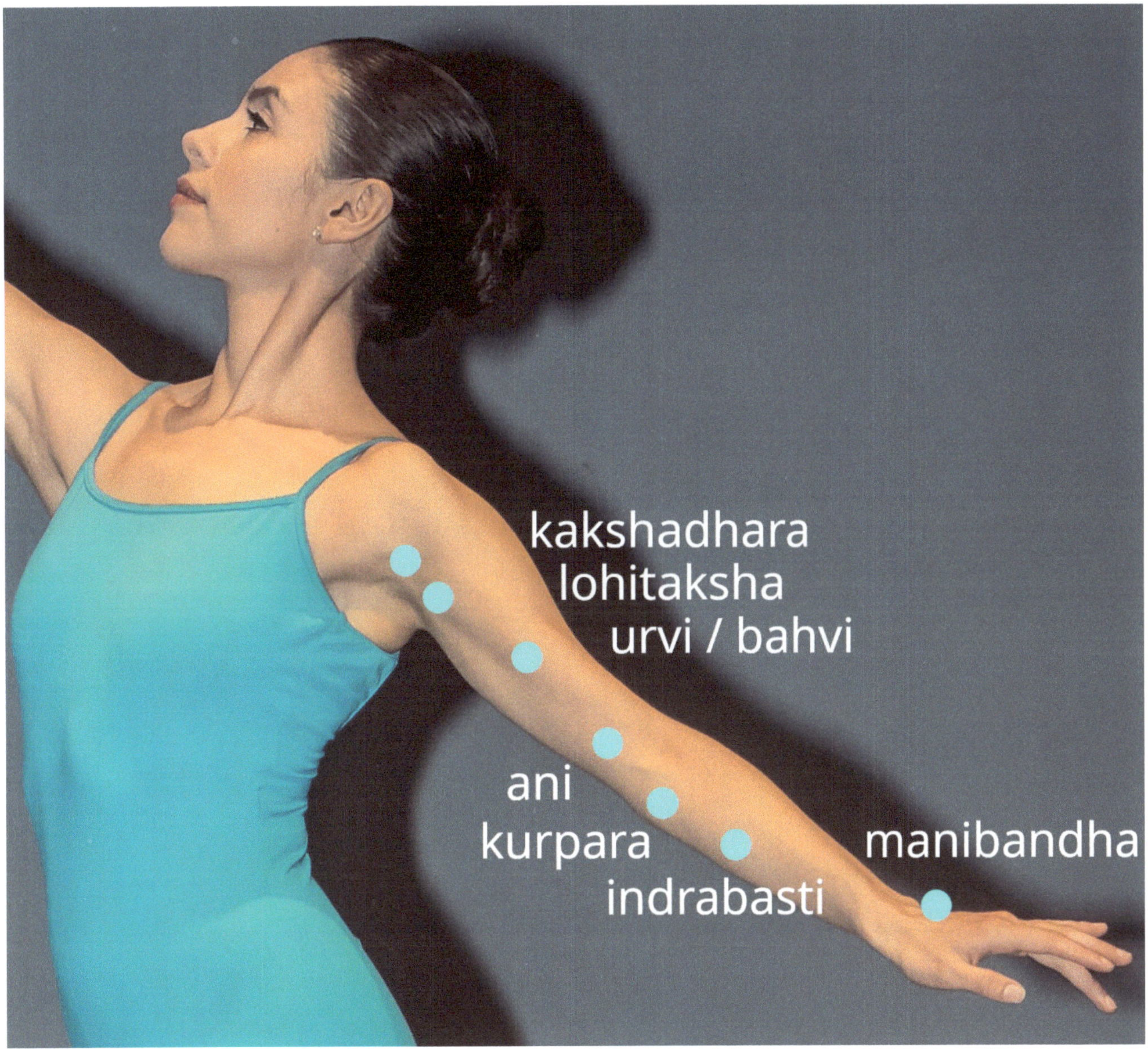

43,44. Kakshadhara Features

A	Name	कक्षधर kakṣadhara (kakshadhara)
B	Marma No. No of Points	43,44. Two
C	Body Part	armpit
D	Precise Location	between armpit and shoulder
E	Tissue Type	स्नायु snāyu (Nerve/Tendon)
F	Size	अर्ध-अङ्गुल ½ angula.
G	Severity	vaikalyakara = long term restlessness
H	Physics/Chemistry	Spring.
I	Chikitsa recommended	Touch lightly with Index finger tip. May do a slow roll of fingertip.
J	Oil recommended	Rose Scent Oil. Simply pour a drop.
K	Meditation / Yogasana	Arm Rotation. Swimming.

kakshadhara, lohitaksha

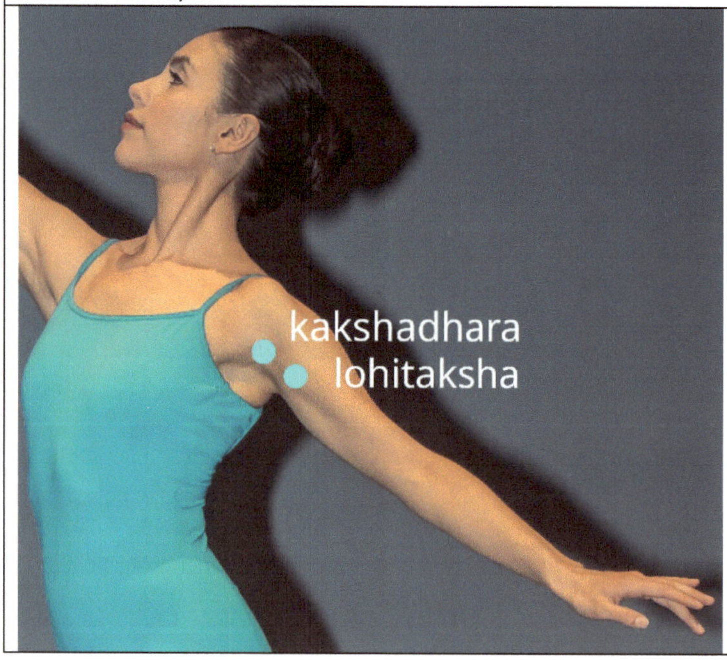

41,42. Lohitaksha Arm Features

A	Name	लोहिताक्ष lohitākṣa (lohitaksha)
B	Marma No. No of Points	41.42. Two
C	Body Part	Arm
D	Precise Location	in the junction at root of arm
E	Tissue Type	सिरा sirā (Tube)
F	Size	अर्ध-अङ्गुल ½ angula.
G	Severity	vaikalyakara = long term restlessness
H	Physics/Chemistry	Spring.
I	Chikitsa recommended	Touch lightly with Index finger tip. May do a slow roll of fingertip.
J	Oil recommended	Rose Scent Oil. Simply pour a drop.
K	Meditation / Yogasana	Arm Rotation. Swimming.

39,40. Urvi Arm Features

A	Name	ऊर्वी (उर्वी) / बाह्वी ūrvī (urvi), bāhvī
B	Marma No. No of Points	107. 1
C	Body Part	Upper arm
D	Precise Location	Center of upper arm
E	Tissue Type	सिरा sirā (Tube)
F	Size	अङ्गुल 1 angula.
G	Severity	vaikalyakara = long term restlessness
H	Physics/Chemistry	Commitment. Long term relationships.
I	Chikitsa recommended	Touch lightly with Index finger tip. May do a slow roll of fingertip.
J	Oil recommended	Kshirabala.
K	Meditation / Yogasana	Arm Rotation. Dumbbells. Swimming.

urvi, ani

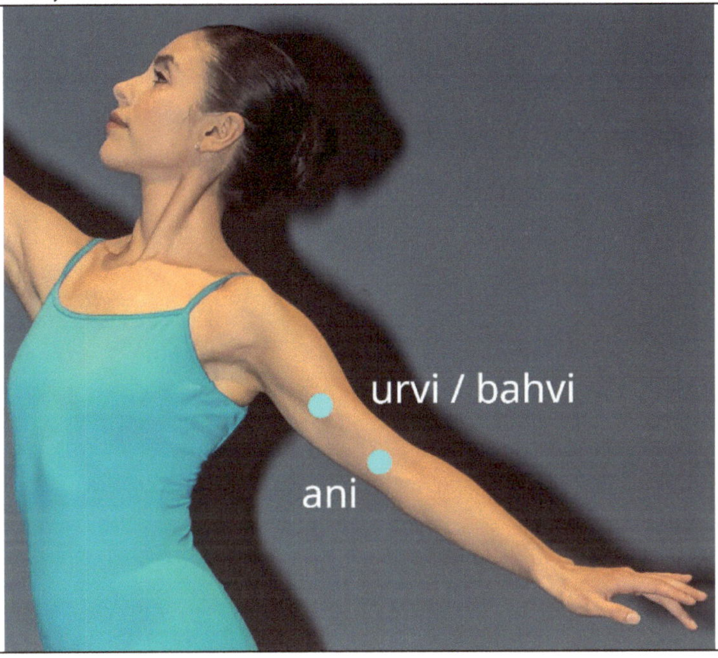

37,38. Ani Arm Features

A	Name	आणि āṇi (ani)
B	Marma No. No of Points	37,38. 1
C	Body Part	Upper arm
D	Precise Location	2 angula above elbow
E	Tissue Type	स्नायु snāyu (Nerve/Tendon)
F	Size	अर्ध-अङ्गुल ½ angula.
G	Severity	vaikalyakara = long term restlessness
H	Physics/Chemistry	Commitment. Long term relationships.
I	Chikitsa recommended	Touch lightly with Index finger tip. May do a slow roll of fingertip.
J	Oil recommended	Kshirabala.
K	Meditation / Yogasana	Arm Rotation. Dumbbells. Swimming.

35,36. Kurpara Features

A	Name	कूर्पर kūrpara (kurpara)
B	Marma No. No of Points	35,36. Two
C	Body Part	Elbow
D	Precise Location	Elbow joint where it touches forearm
E	Tissue Type	सन्धि-मर्म Joint.
F	Size	त्रि-अङ्गुल 3 angula.
G	Severity	vaikalyakara = long term restlessness
H	Physics/Chemistry	Cheerfulness.
I	Chikitsa recommended	Hold tightly with arc of thumb and forefinger
J	Oil recommended	Ashwagandha. Mahanarayana.
K	Meditation / Yogasana	Arm Rotation. Dumbbells.

kurpara, indrabasti

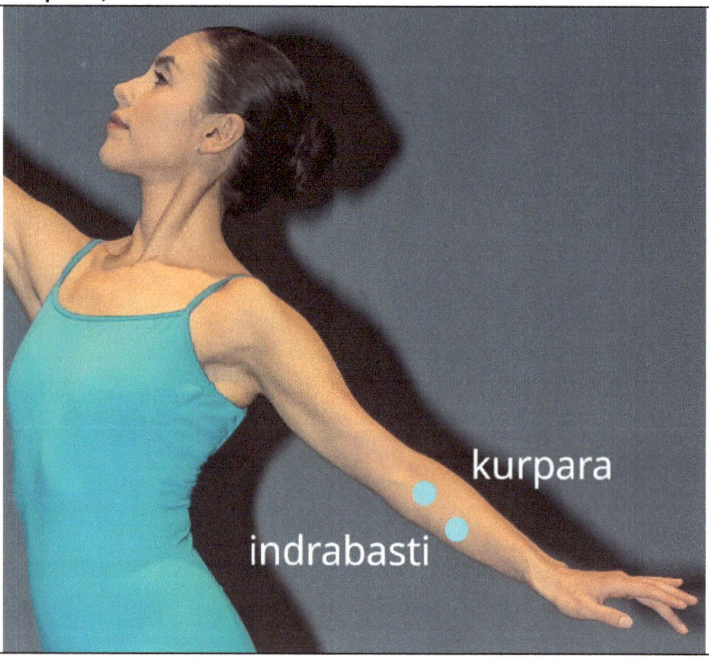

33,34. Indrabasti Arm Features

A	Name	इन्द्रबस्ति indrabasti
B	Marma No. No of Points	33,34. Two
C	Body Part	Forearm
D	Precise Location	Midpoint of forearm
E	Tissue Type	मांस māṃsa (Muscle)
F	Size	अर्ध-अङ्गुल ½ angula.
G	Severity	kālāntaraprāṇahara = fatal after a while
H	Physics/Chemistry	Youthfulness
I	Chikitsa recommended	Touch lightly with Index finger tip. May do a slow roll of fingertip.
J	Oil recommended	Kshirabala.
K	Meditation / Yogasana	Arm Rotation. Dumbbells.

31,32. Manibandha Features

A	Name	मणिबन्ध maṇibandha (manibandha)
B	Marma No. No of Points	31,32. Two
C	Body Part	Wrist
D	Precise Location	Edge of wrist bone towards hand
E	Tissue Type	सन्धि-मर्म Sandhi Joint.
F	Size	द्वि-अङ्गुल 2 angula.
G	Severity	rujākara = intense pain
H	Physics/Chemistry	Cheerfulness.
I	Chikitsa recommended	Hold tightly with arc of thumb and forefinger
J	Oil recommended	Ashwagandha. Mahanarayana.
K	Meditation / Yogasana	Wrist Rotation. Dumbbells. Swimming.

manibandha

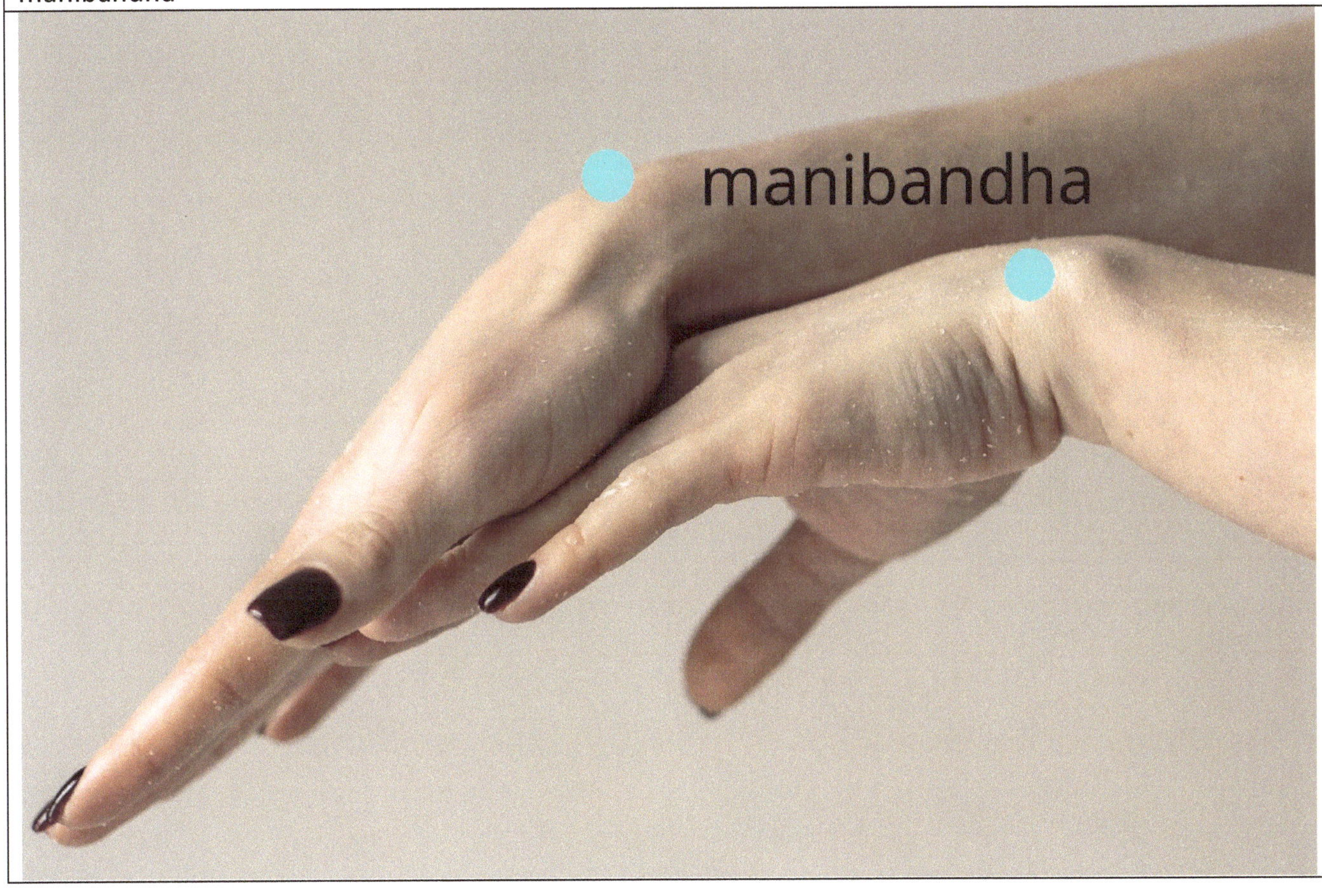

Pair Points in Hands = 4x2 = 8

KurchaShira hand	2	Extend the thumb till it joins the wrist
Kurcha hand	2	thumb base
TalaHridaya hand	2	palm center
Kshipra hand	2	V junction between thumb and index finger
Points subTotal	**8**	

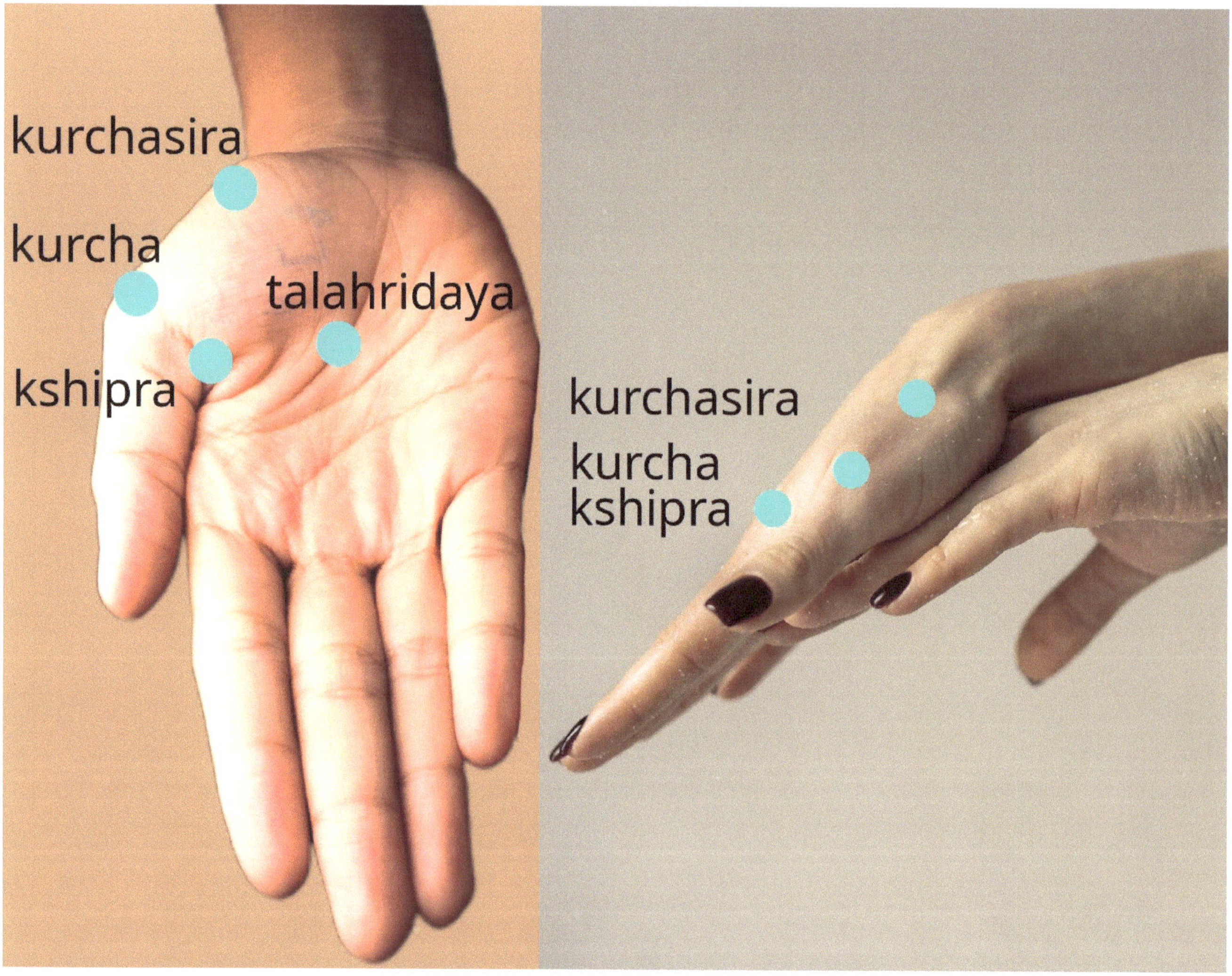

29,30. Kurchashira Hand Features

A	Name	कूर्चशिर kūrcaśira (kurchashira)
B	Marma No. No of Points	29,30. Two
C	Body Part	Hand
D	Precise Location	Extend the thumb till it touches the wrist
E	Tissue Type	स्नायु snāyu (Nerve/Tendon)
F	Size	अङ्गुल 1 angula.
G	Severity	rujākara = intense pain
H	Physics/Chemistry	Decision Making.
I	Chikitsa recommended	Touch lightly with Index finger tip. May do a slow roll of fingertip.
J	Oil recommended	Shakti drops. Simply pour a drop.
K	Meditation / Yogasana	Rotating and stretching the thumb. Flexing the Palms.

kurchashira, kurcha

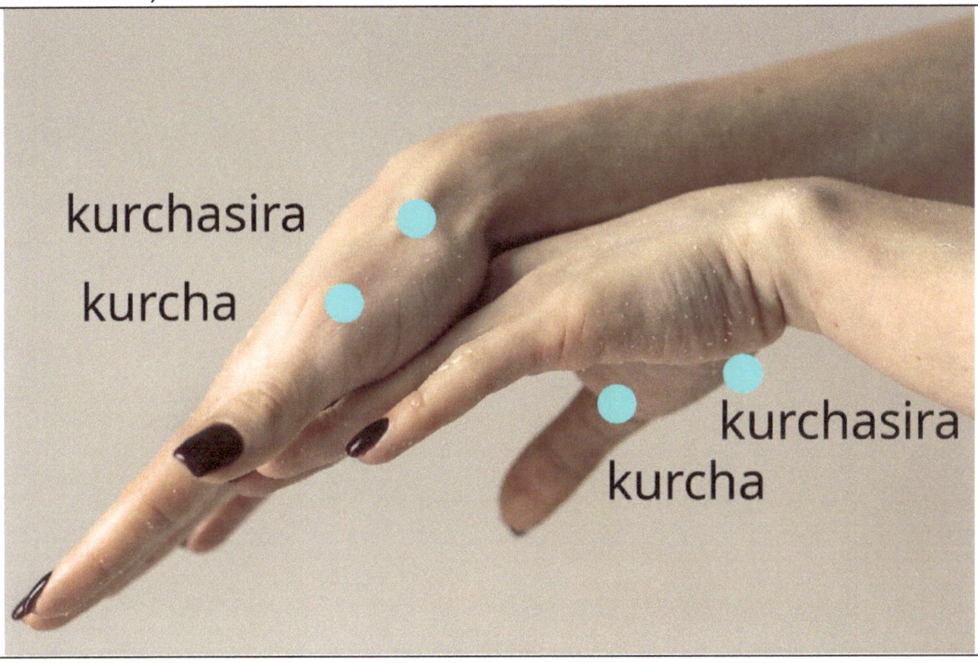

27,28. Kurcha Hand Features

A	Name	कूर्च kūrca (kurcha)
B	Marma No. No of Points	27,28. Two
C	Body Part	Hand
D	Precise Location	base of thumb
E	Tissue Type	स्नायु snāyu (Nerve/Tendon)
F	Size	पाणितल palm
G	Severity	vaikalyakara = long term restlessness
H	Physics/Chemistry	Youthfulness.
I	Chikitsa recommended	Touch lightly with cupped palm. May keep the palm at a slight gap.
J	Oil recommended	Shakti drops. Simply pour a drop.
K	Meditation / Yogasana	Rotating and stretching the thumb. Flexing the Palms.

25,26. Talahridaya Hand Features

A	Name	तलहृदय talahṛdaya (talahridaya)
B	Marma No. No of Points	25,26. Two
C	Body Part	palm
D	Precise Location	Exact center of palm, directly in line with middle finger.
E	Tissue Type	मांस māṃsa (Muscle)
F	Size	अर्ध-अङ्गुल ½ angula.
G	Severity	kālāntaraprāṇahara = fatal after a while
H	Physics/Chemistry	Youthfulness
I	Chikitsa recommended	Touch lightly with Index finger tip. May do a slow roll of fingertip.
J	Oil recommended	Mustard Oil.
K	Meditation / Yogasana	Massage the palm and clap well

talahridaya, kshipra

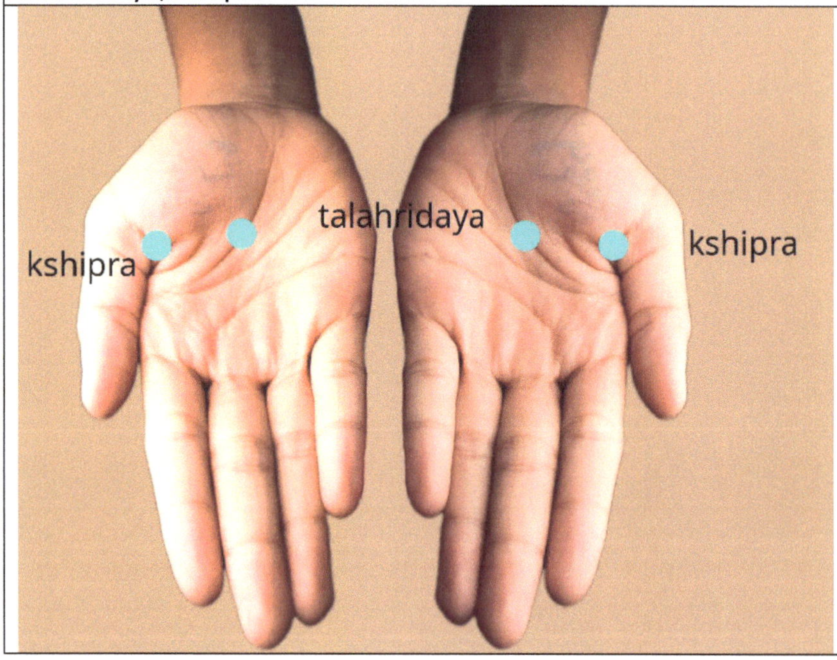

23,24. Kshipra Hand Features

A	Name	क्षिप्र kṣipra (kshipra)
B	Marma No. No of Points	23,24. Two
C	Body Part	Between Thumb and index finger
D	Precise Location	V junction where they join the hand
E	Tissue Type	स्नायु snāyu (Nerve/Tendon)
F	Size	अर्ध-अङ्गुल ½ angula.
G	Severity	kālāntaraprāṇahara = fatal after a while
H	Physics/Chemistry	Speed of decision making
I	Chikitsa recommended	Touch firmly with Index finger tip. May do a slow roll of fingertip.
J	Oil recommended	Mustard Oil.
K	Meditation / Yogasana	Massage the palm and clap well

Pair Points at Genitals = 2x2 = 4

Vitapa		2	Perineum between anus and scrotum Male/vulva Female	
Lohitaksha leg		2	Where thigh meets torso	
Points subTotal		**4**		
Additional Chikitsa Points (not shown)				
	Vrushna		Male	On the balls
	Yoni Oshtha		Female	Either side of vulva

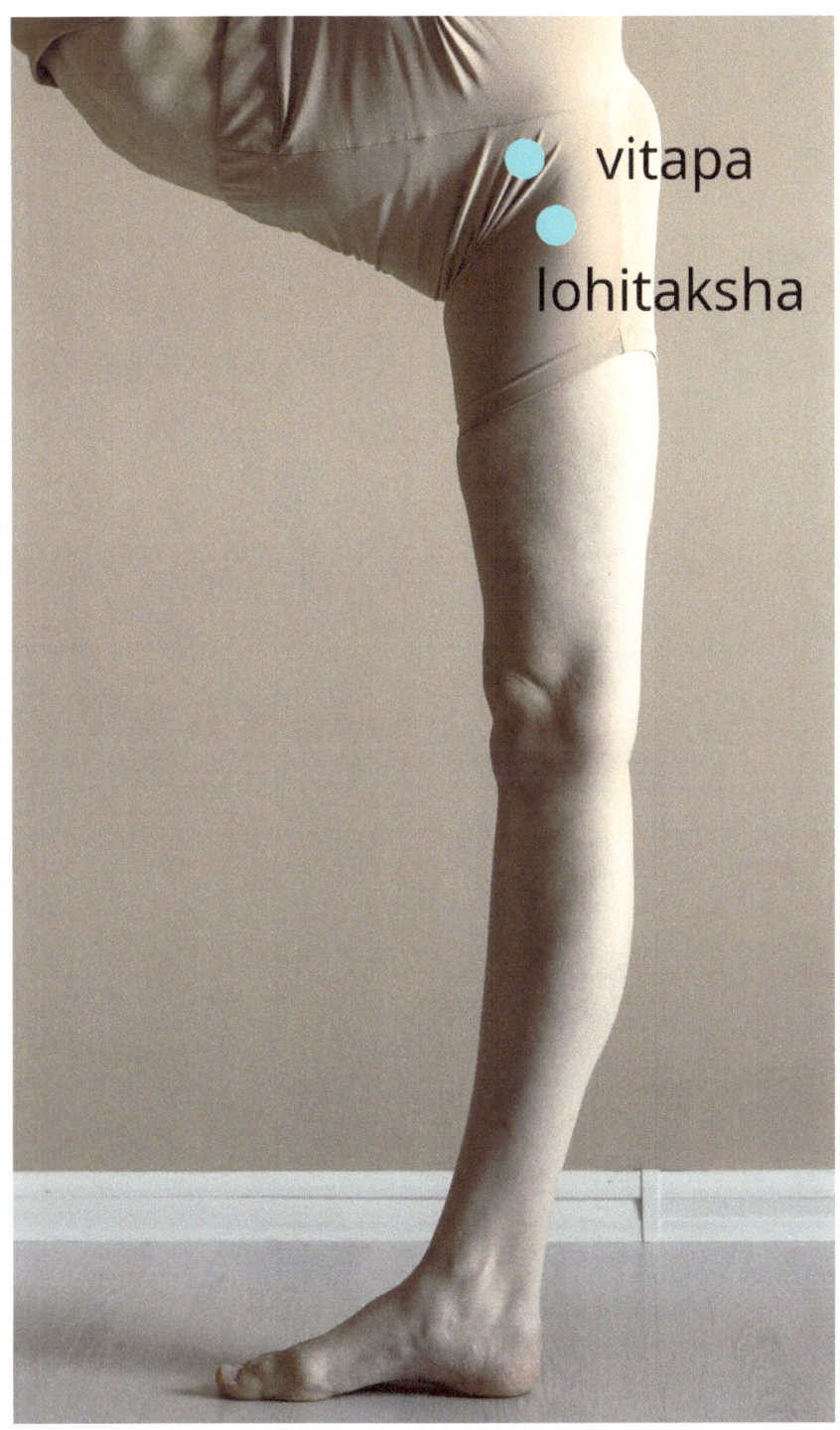

21,22. Vitapa Features

A	Name	विटप viṭapa (vitapa)
B	Marma No. No of Points	21,22. Two
C	Body Part	Genitals
D	Precise Location	between the inguinal canal and scrotum
E	Tissue Type	स्नायु snāyu (Nerve/Tendon)
F	Size	अर्ध-अङ्गुल ½ angula.
G	Severity	vaikalyakara = long term restlessness
H	Physics/Chemistry	Spring.
I	Chikitsa recommended	Simply give instructions to take attention there.
J	Oil recommended	Fresh Cream. Rose Scent Oil.
K	Meditation / Yogasana	Hari Om Meditation. Ashwini Mudra. Moolabandha.

vitapa, lohitaksha

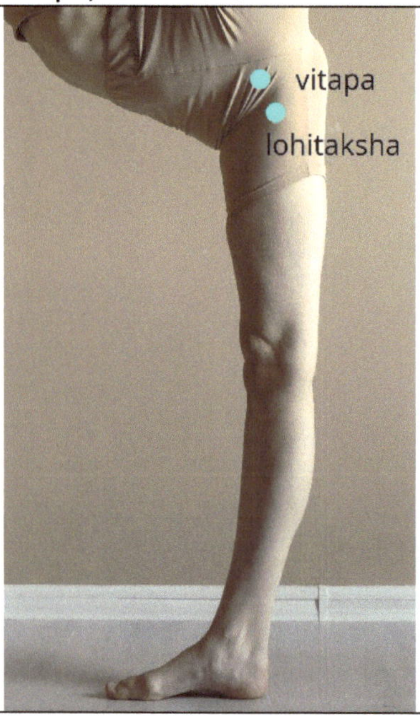

19,20. Lohitaksha Leg Features

A	Name	लोहिताक्ष lohitākṣa (lohitaksha)
B	Marma No. No of Points	19,20. Two
C	Body Part	Genitals
D	Precise Location	in the groin junction at root of thigh
E	Tissue Type	सिरा sirā (Tube)
F	Size	अर्ध-अङ्गुल ½ angula.
G	Severity	vaikalyakara = long term restlessness
H	Physics/Chemistry	Spring.
I	Chikitsa recommended	Simply give instructions to take attention there
J	Oil recommended	Fresh Cream. Rose Scent Oil.
K	Meditation / Yogasana	Leg lifts. Leg Rotation. Swimming.

Pair Points in Legs = 5x2 = 10

Urvi leg	2	thigh midpoint
Ani leg	2	lower part of upper leg
Janu	2	knee joint
Indrabasti leg	2	lower leg calf center
Gulpha	2	ankle
Points subTotal	**10**	

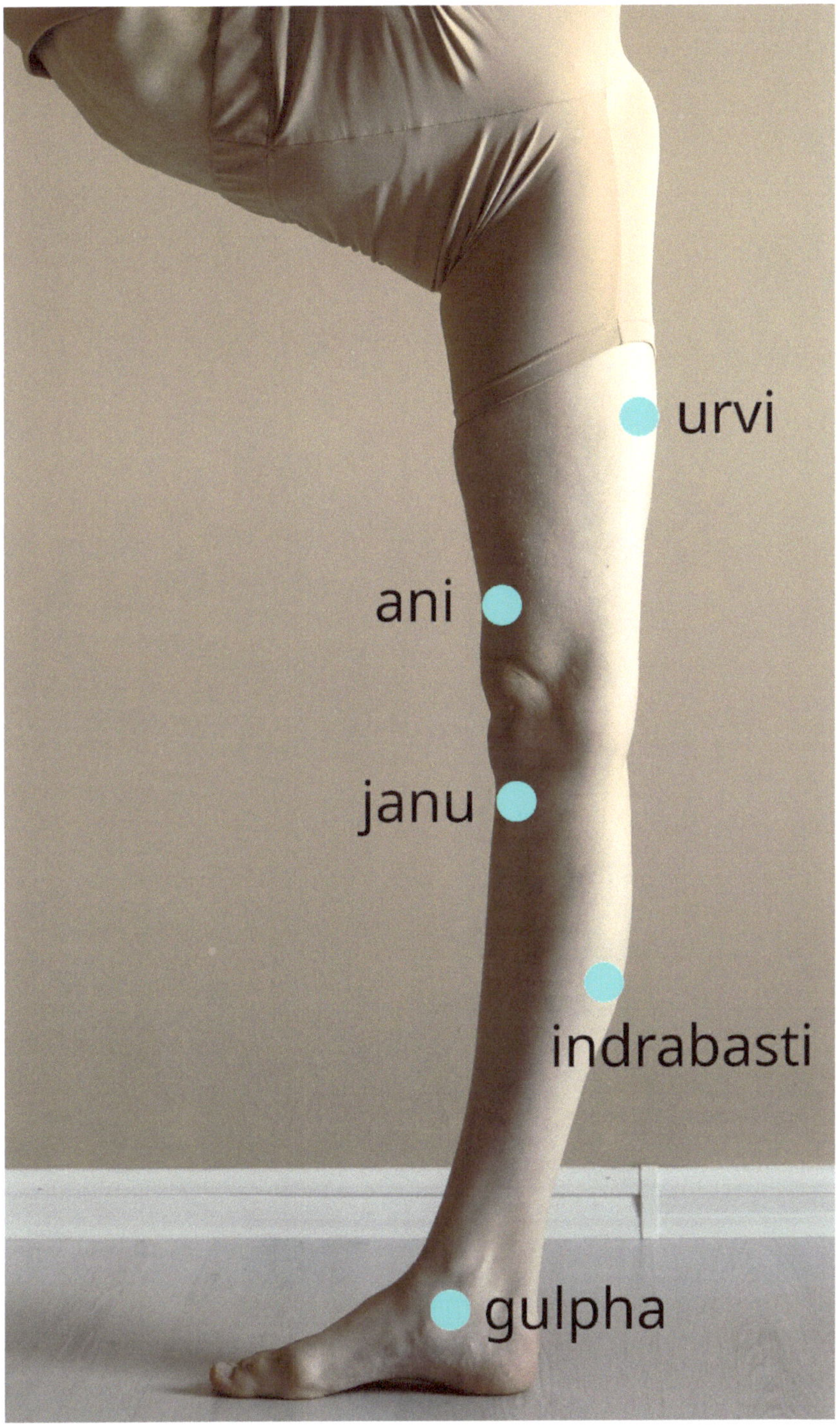

17,18. Urvi Leg Features

A	Name	ऊर्वी ūrvī (urvi)
B	Marma No. No of Points	17,18. Two
C	Body Part	Thigh
D	Precise Location	Center of thigh
E	Tissue Type	सिरा sirā (Tube)
F	Size	अङ्गुल 1 angula.
G	Severity	vaikalyakara = long term restlessness
H	Physics/Chemistry	Commitment. Long term relationships.
I	Chikitsa recommended	Touch lightly with Index finger tip. May do a slow roll of fingertip.
J	Oil recommended	Kshirabala.
K	Meditation / Yogasana	Butterfly. Swimming. Massaging the thigh muscles slowly.

urvi, ani

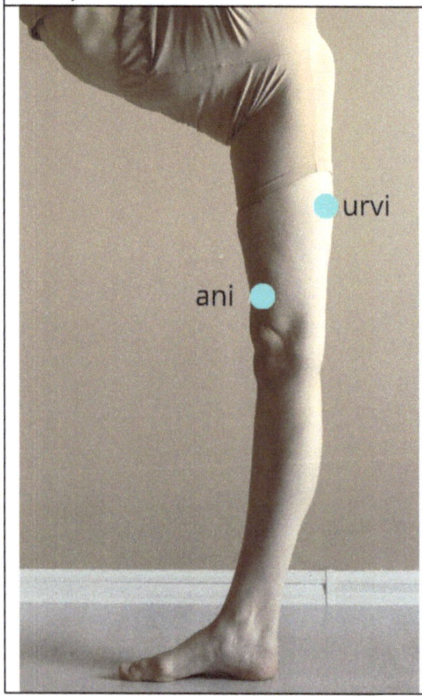

15,16. Ani Leg Features

A	Name	आणि āṇi (ani)
B	Marma No. No of Points	15,16. Two
C	Body Part	Upper leg
D	Precise Location	2 angula above knee
E	Tissue Type	स्नायु snāyu (Nerve/Tendon)
F	Size	अर्ध-अङ्गुल ½ angula.
G	Severity	vaikalyakara = long term restlessness
H	Physics/Chemistry	Commitment. Long term relationships.
I	Chikitsa recommended	Touch lightly with Index finger tip. May do a slow roll of fingertip.
J	Oil recommended	Kshirabala.
K	Meditation / Yogasana	Paschimottanasana. Sarvangasana. Stretching the knee muscles.

13,14. Janu Features

A	Name	जानु jānu (janu)
B	Marma No. No of Points	13,14. Two
C	Body Part	Knee
D	Precise Location	Knee joint where it touches lower leg
E	Tissue Type	सन्धि-मर्म Joint.
F	Size	त्रि-अङ्गुल 3 angula.
G	Severity	vaikalyakara = long term restlessness
H	Physics/Chemistry	Cheerfulness.
I	Chikitsa recommended	Hold tightly with arc of thumb and forefinger
J	Oil recommended	Ashwangandha. Mahanarayana.
K	Meditation / Yogasana	Paschimottanasana. Sarvangasana. Flexing the knee muscles.

janu, indrabasti

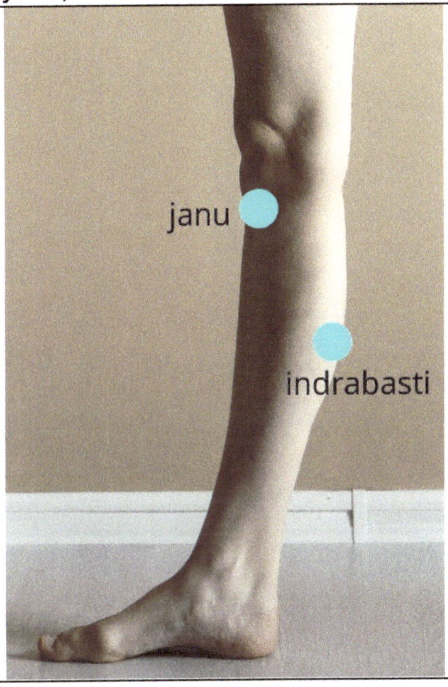

11,12. Indrabasti Leg Features

A	Name	इन्द्रबस्ति indrabasti
B	Marma No. No of Points	11,12. Two
C	Body Part	Lower Leg
D	Precise Location	Midpoint of calf, that pumps back and recirculates blood
E	Tissue Type	मांस māṃsa (Muscle)
F	Size	अर्ध-अङ्गुल ½ angula.
G	Severity	kālāntaraprāṇahara = fatal after a while
H	Physics/Chemistry	Youthfulness
I	Chikitsa recommended	Touch lightly with Index finger tip. May do a slow roll of fingertip.
J	Oil recommended	Kshirabala.
K	Meditation / Yogasana	Janushirshasana.

9,10. Gulpha Features

A	Name	गुल्फ gulpha
B	Marma No. No of Points	9,10. Two
C	Body Part	Ankle
D	Precise Location	At lower edge of ankle bone
E	Tissue Type	सन्धि-मर्म Joint.
F	Size	द्वि-अङ्गुल 2 angula.
G	Severity	rujākara = intense pain
H	Physics/Chemistry	Cheerfulness.
I	Chikitsa recommended	Hold tightly with arc of thumb and forefinger
J	Oil recommended	Ashwangandha. Mahanarayana.
K	Meditation / Yogasana	Ankle Rotation. Standing on heels and toes alternately.

gulpha

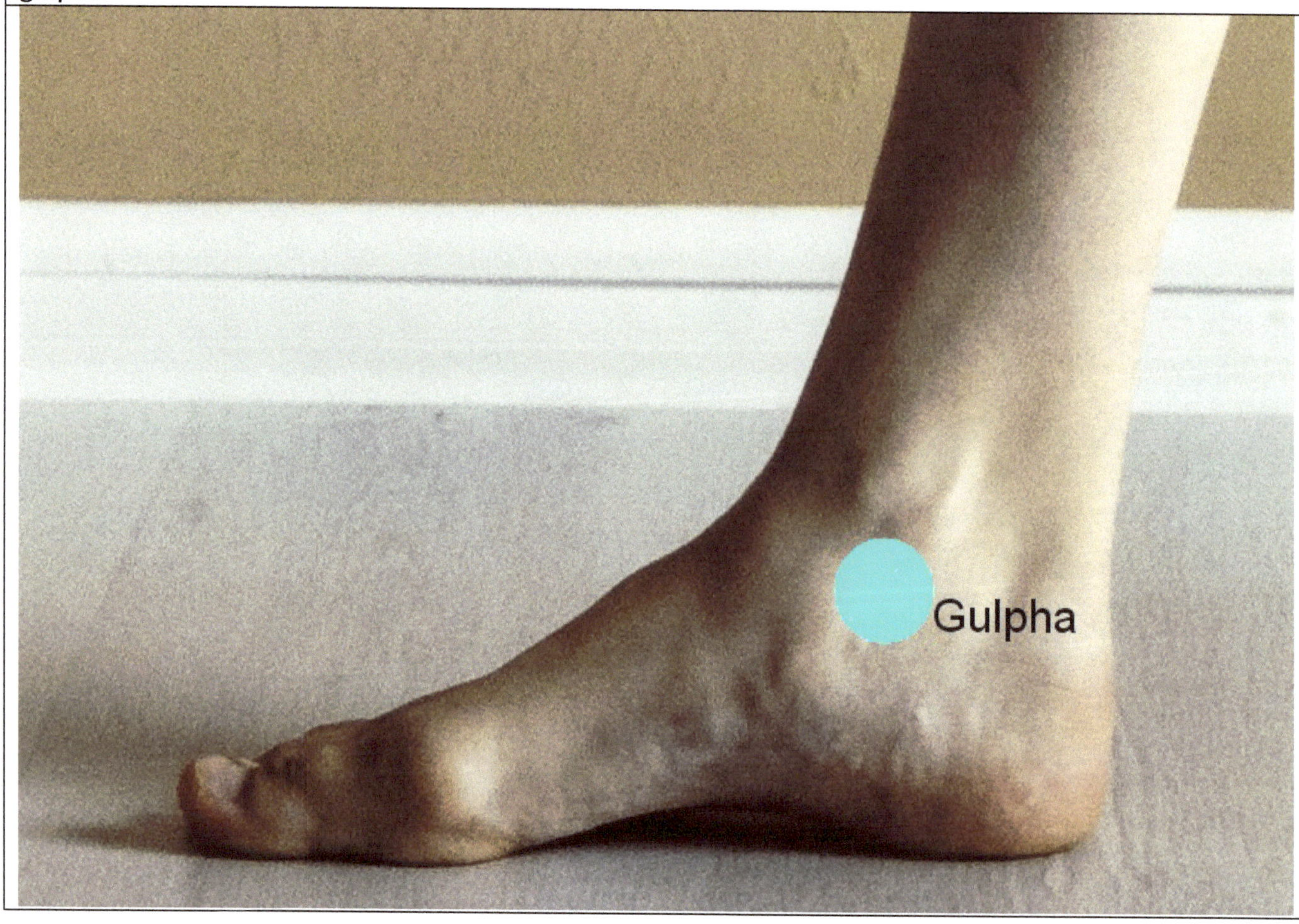

Pair Points in Feet = 4x2 = 8

KurchaShira foot	2	Extend the big toe till where it joins the leg
Kurcha foot	2	base of big toe
TalaHridaya foot	2	sole center
Kshipra foot	2	between big toe and second toe finger
Points subTotal	**8**	

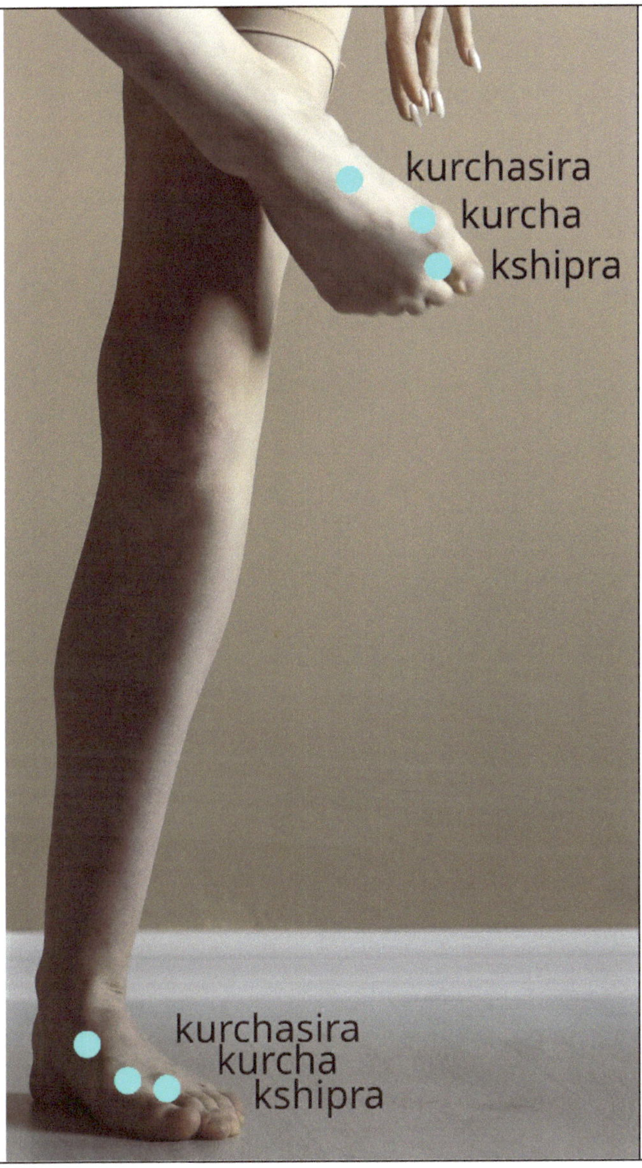

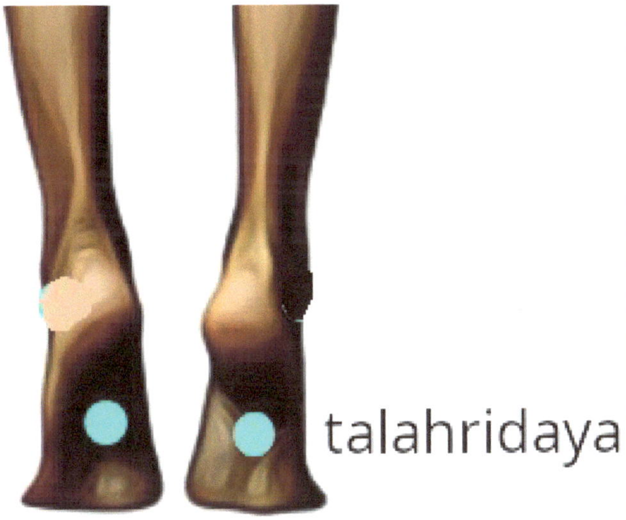

7,8. Kurchashira Feet Features

A	Name	कूर्चशिर kūrcaśira (kurchashira)
B	Marma No. No of Points	7,8. Two
C	Body Part	Foot
D	Precise Location	Extend the big toe till it touches the leg
E	Tissue Type	स्नायु snāyu (Nerve/Tendon)
F	Size	अङ्गुल 1 angula.
G	Severity	rujākara = intense pain
H	Physics/Chemistry	Decision Making.
I	Chikitsa recommended	Touch lightly with Index finger tip. May do a slow roll of fingertip.
J	Oil recommended	Shakti drops. Simply pour a drop.
K	Meditation / Yogasana	Rotating and stretching the toes. Flexing the soles.

Kurchashira, kurcha

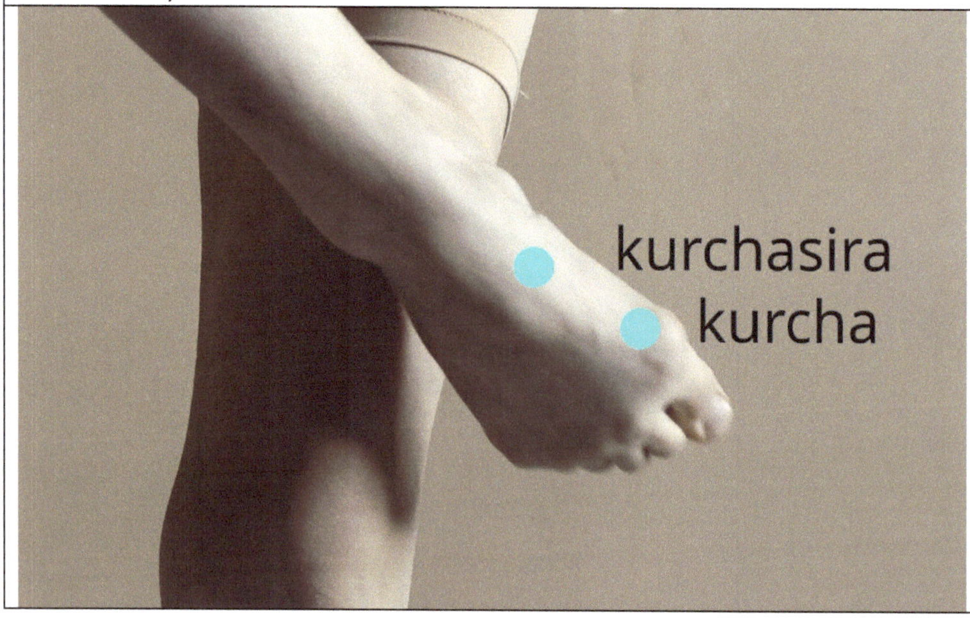

5,6. Kurcha Feet Features

A	Name	कूर्च kūrca (kurcha)
B	Marma No. No of Points	5,6. Two
C	Body Part	Foot
D	Precise Location	base of big toe
E	Tissue Type	स्नायु snāyu (Nerve/Tendon)
F	Size	पाणितल palm
G	Severity	vaikalyakara = long term restlessness
H	Physics/Chemistry	Decision Making.
I	Chikitsa recommended	Touch lightly with cupped palm. May keep the palm at a slight gap.
J	Oil recommended	Shakti drops. Simply pour a drop.
K	Meditation / Yogasana	Rotating and stretching the toes. Flexing the soles.

3,4. Talahridaya Feet Features

A	Name	तलहृदय talahṛdaya (talahridaya)
B	Marma No. No of Points	3,4. Two
C	Body Part	Sole of foot
D	Precise Location	Exact center of sole, directly in line with middle toe.
E	Tissue Type	māṃsa (Muscle)
F	Size	½ angula
G	Severity	kālāntaraprāṇahara = fatal after a while
H	Physics/Chemistry	Youthfulness
I	Chikitsa recommended	Touch firmly with Index finger tip. May do a slow roll of fingertip.
J	Oil recommended	Mustard Oil.
K	Meditation / Yogasana	Massage the soles thoroughly

talahridaya, kshipra

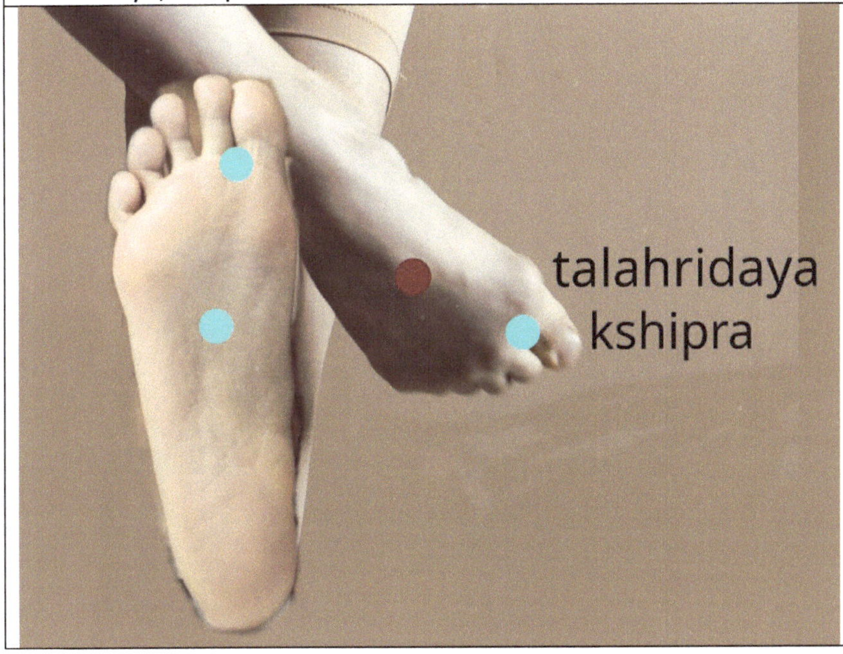

1,2. Kshipra Feet Features

A	Name	क्षिप्र kṣipra (kshipra)
B	Marma No. No of Points	1,2. Two
C	Body Part	Between Big toe and adjacent toe finger
D	Precise Location	junction of these two toes where they join the foot
E	Tissue Type	snāyu (Nerve/Tendon)
F	Size	½ angula
G	Severity	kālāntaraprāṇahara = fatal after a while
H	Physics/Chemistry	Speed of decision making
I	Chikitsa recommended	Touch firmly with Index finger tip. May do a slow roll of fingertip.
J	Oil recommended	Mustard Oil.
K	Meditation / Yogasana	Rotating and stretching the toes.

Glowing Body and Consciousness

Our body is made of threads of light, weaved to a perfection. At times, due to our lifestyle, demands, cravings and pressures, these light threads undergo imperfections of three types:

- the length of a thread ray gets shortened or elongated
- the amplitude of a light beam gets under or over normal
- the light ray diverges outside or gets diffracted unevenly

Marma Chikitsa comes in here to restore the original light thread. By a simple touch at a Marma point, the innate consciousness resurfaces there and the thread of the body fabric gets healed.

Marma Chikitsa is a combination of the following methods:

- light touch at a Marma point with finger or palm
- medium pressure on the Marma point
- deep massage on the Marma point
- a suggestion from a distance without touching
- pouring a drop of aromatic oil on the Marma point
- giving a tender kiss on the Marma point
- using a soft teakwood pencil for touch
- using a well fashioned brass or silver tool for touch
- using gentle instrumental music
- affirmative auto suggestions for the brain to absorb

Bioluminescent Body and Marma

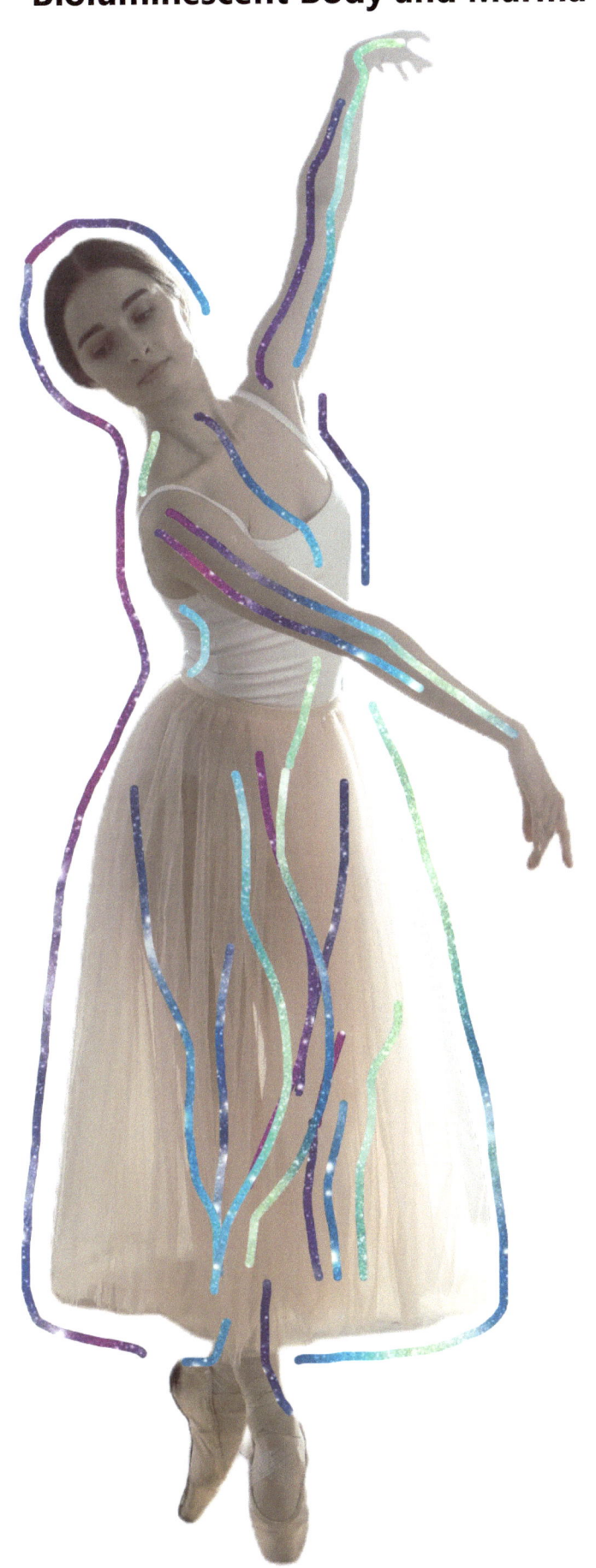

Simply Effective Marma Therapy techniques

Some of these practices you are already doing.

Many of these you are certainly aware of.

Now is the time
Now is the chance
Now one can put in the effort

for a method that your heart is willing to do and so is your faith...

Barefoot Walking

Walking barefoot on the lawn. Walking bare feet on a sandy beach.

Oiled Clapping

Pour a spoonful of Mustard Oil (sarson) on your palms and start clapping vigorously. Continue for 20 minutes. Now clap on the edges of the hands and make body movements as well. Continue for 5 minutes. Then become still. Observe your breath. Give thanks for this moment. And it's done.

Boisterous Laughter

You will need to listen to a ticklish joke from a family member or the internet. When laughter comes, just erupt, do not hold back. After 10 minutes of boisterous laughter, calm down and slowly stop. Then become still. Observe your breath. Give thanks for this moment. And it's done.

Eating together

Call all the family members to the dinner table, and serve everyone properly. Then with a group prayer, begin to eat. Allow the conversation to flow if any, however not regarding any bitterness or grievance. When you are done, help in serving and clearing the table. Then become still. Observe your breath. Give thanks for this moment. And it's done.

Guided Meditation

A guided meditation by Guruji is one of the most effective marma techniques.

Yoganidra

Yoganidra is a subtle marma practice that works wonders.

Showering Properly

Having a really good shower with touching/scrubbing all parts thoroughly.

Dipping feet in lukewarm water with Rocksalt

Fill a bucket with lukewarm water and add a tablespoon of Himalayan Pink Salt. Sit comfortably dipping your feet until the knees.

Palming the Eyes

Palming the eyes for 20 minutes.

Shirodhara and Abhyanga Panchakarma

Having a session of Shirodhara coupled with Abhyanga panchakarma massage.

Mountain Trekking

Going for a long trek in the hills or the woods is what energizes and activates all the Marma points.

Listening to a Rudram Chant

Listening to powerful Vedic chants like the Rudri, Om Namah Shivaya, Gayatri Mantra etc. activates the Marma points.

Applying Henna Mehandi

Applying mehndi to the hands and feet during festivals and cultural events is a common practice by girls to energize the Marma points.

A traditional Marma Chikitsa Protocol

Our Marma Therapy Protocol consists of a Polarity Routine followed by a Touch Routine. Takes 45-55 minutes from start to finish. It is based on personal cleanliness, regular sadhana, observing a vegetarian diet, and following the Patanjali principles of Yama and Niyama. Here is a simple technique, however all key steps should be **learnt in person** from a qualified trainer. In some cases, the opposite part of limb gives a support during Marma Therapy. The Touch must be gentle, caring, sober.

Disclaimer – What follows is just a general guideline for established practitioners to refer to.

-1. Be regular in your Sadhana, Satsang and Guru Puja.

---

0. Inform the Client of having a light stomach, taking a fresh shower, and wearing a comfortable open-neck dress before arriving. If possible, they may remove hair bands, clips, ornaments, watch etc. before beginning.

---

1. Welcome the Client and make him feel relaxed with a sip of water and use of washroom, and washing face and hands and feet.

---

2. See that the therapy room is relatively noise free and interruption free. Lighting is decent and gadgets are switched off. A conveniently positioned wall clock or table clock with seconds hand is necessary.
3. The chikitsa can be done on a bedded cot or on a mattress laid on the floor. Arrange the same as per mutual convenience. A proper CST Bed or Marma bed can also be arranged or bought. Have a couple of stools (or chairs) positioned at client's head and their right side beforehand.
4. Cover the mattress with two freshly washed bedsheets.

---

5. Ask the Client to lie down comfortably in Shavasana.
6. Gently take your position at the right side of Client, just near their right wrist.
7. Advise that the session will be deeply relaxing, in case of discomfort to let us know, follow simple instructions if any.
8. Locate the Nabhi and Adhipati of Client by self-demonstration since their own angula and palm measurements will be accurate for their body. Now they may close their eyes and be at ease. (adhipati can be located by the client's palm lower edge placed on their 3rd eye, then where their middle finger reaches on the crown is adhipati.

---

9. Gently move to the head side of Client and take few deep breaths.
10. Chant the Dhanvantari prayer.
11. Build a touch rapport with Client by lightly touching their shoulders with tips of fingers.

---

12. Glance at the clock and you are ready to begin!

POLARITY ROUTINE

Ten Stages – At each stage breathe calmly with appropriate light visualization and Japa for 90 sec.

13. Randolph Stone's **i.) Skull hold** is the starting stage.
Gently lift their head a bit and slide your palms underneath their head.
Make the head of the Client rest on your open palms. Your thumb and Index fingers just encircling the ears without touching the ears of Client. Softly give instructions to the Client for keeping awareness at 3rd eye.

14. Polarity **ii.) Skull mirror** with right hand below the head and left hand on the forehead just above eyebrows of Client.

15. Polarity **iii.) Skull midline mirror** with right hand below the head rotated at 90° wrt your left hand, such that your middle finger is aligned to their skull's midline. Left hand stays in position on forehead as in previous stage.

16. Polarity **iv.) Skull pull** with the pulps of your thumbs positioned on sthapani marma point (3rd eye ajna chakra). Palms with fingers widespread below Client's head, but not touching their head. Only the pulps of your fingers are touching the Client's head, with a pressure that is faint, with *an intention* to pull their skull towards you.

---

17. Polarity **v.) Shoulder hard press** (**Amsa**) with both hands' fingers touching Client's shoulders near the neck, press really hard such that a sensation travels to their knee and heels.

---

18. Now you move softly to the right side of Client, near their knees. Position yourself appropriately so your stance and breath are stable without strain. Reestablish your silent Japa.

19. Polarity **vi.) Knee hold** (**Janu**) with your both hands thumb and index finger placed just below Client's knees. Your touch is very gentle. Your thumb and index finger give the appearance of a clock showing 4 O'clock (left hand on left knee) and 8 O'clock (right hand on right knee). After a minute you may release the knee hold and do three swipes with your raised hands in air traveling from their knees towards their feet and beyond.

20. Now you move softly on the right side of Client, near their right foot. We *do not* cross the midline Craniocaudal axis of Client. We remain to the right side of the Client's Sagittal plane. Position yourself appropriately so your stance and breath are stable without strain.

21. Polarity **vii.) Ankle hold** (**Gulpha**) with your thumb and index finger placed just below Client's ankle bone. Your touch is very gentle. Both hands as in previous stage. Release the hold and do a single swipe.

22. Now move and gently take your position at the right side of Client, just near their right wrist.

23. Polarity **viii-a.) Nabhi mirror** with your right hand below and left palm positioned just below Client's nabhi. Roll up the top bedspread and lift it so that your right hand can easily slide and be positioned under Client's back just above their waist. Softly give instructions to Client for keeping awareness at manipura chakra and internal organs there.

24. Now you move softly on the right side of Client, near their neck. Position yourself appropriately so your stance and breath are stable without strain.

25. Polarity **viii-b.) Upper Sternum mirror** with your right hand below and left palm positioned just below Client's clavicle. Roll up the top bedspread and lift it so that your right hand can easily slide and be positioned under Client's back just below their neck. Softly give instructions to Client for keeping awareness at anahata chakra and internal organs there. Our left palm is placed on the *Manubrium breast bone* of the Client, and the right palm is mirrored below their back.

26. Now position yourself appropriately so your stance and breath are stable without strain. Reestablish your silent Japa.

27. Polarity **ix-a.) Left hip bone rock** with your right hand firmly placed. First position your left hand on Client's *right* shoulder and push hard so that a diagonal is observed on Client's torso. Now place right hand firmly on *left* hip bone of Client and rock *left* hip bone at a gentle pace.

28. Polarity **ix-b.) Right hip bone rock** with your right hand firmly placed. First position your left hand on Client's *left* shoulder and push hard so that a diagonal is observed on Client's torso. Now place right hand firmly on *right* hip bone of Client and rock *right* hip bone at a gentle pace.

29. Now position yourself appropriately so your stance and breath are stable without strain.

30. Polarity **x.) Nabhi rock** with your right hand firmly placed just below Client's navel. First position your left hand on Client's forehead just above their eyebrows. Now place right hand firmly just below Client's navel and rock it at a gentle pace.

Here ends the ten stage polarity routine. Breathe calmly and reestablish your silent Japa.

Changeover using YOUTH MUDRA

31. Now gently move to the head side of Client and take few deep breaths.
32. Make both hands in Youth Mudra (for each hand, curl index finger to touch midline of thumb) . Place your right middle finger on sthapani marma point (3rd eye ajna chakra) of Client. Apply gentle pressure. Place your left middle finger on adhipati marma point (top of the head sahasrara chakra) of Client. Apply gentle pressure. Hold for 90 sec and release.

Note: This is the only stage where the right hand is above and the left hand is below. In all other stages, the right hand was below and the left hand was above.

TOUCH ROUTINE

5 Head Stages
4 Eye Stages
4 Nose+Lips Stages
4 Cheek+Ear Stages
3 Neck + 3 Throat Stages
4 Chest+Abdomen Midline Stages
At each stage breathe calmly with appropriate visualization and Japa for half a minute.

5 Head Stages
33. Touch **i.) Manyamula (Simanta5) marma point** touch with your right index finger and roll the Client's skin there clockwise at an easy pace. For ease in accessing the point, gently lift and turn client's head to the left a bit.
34. Touch **ii.) Shivarandhra (Simanta4) marma point** (shikha of the head where ponytail is made) touch with your right index finger and roll the Client's skin there clockwise at an easy pace.
35. Touch **iii.) Adhipati (Brahmarandhra) marma point** (top of the head sahasrara chakra Brahmarandhra) touch with your right index finger and roll the Client's skin there clockwise at an easy pace.
36. Touch **iv.) Vishnurandhra (Simanta3) marma point** (two angula towards the forehead wrt adhipati marma point)touch with your right index finger and roll the Client's skin there clockwise at an easy pace.
37. Touch **v.) Sthapani marma point** touch with your right index finger and roll the Client's skin there clockwise at an easy pace.

Note: In popular textbooks the Adhipati marma point is named Vishnurandhra. However, the ideal name is Brahmarandhra as given here. Consequently, the name of the marma point two angula towards the forehead is also changed here from that seen in standard marma books.

---

4 Eye Stages
38. Touch **i.) Bhruh Antara marma points pair** (**Shringataka eyes extended)** (inner side of both eyebrows) touch and PULL with both thumbs angled.
39. Touch **ii.) Kaninaka marma points pair (Shringataka eyes)** (inner side of both eyes) PUSH gently with both index fingers inclined at 45°.
40. Touch **iii.) Apanga marma points pair** (depression at outer edge of both eyes) PRESS gently with both index fingers.
41. Touch **iv.) Avarta marma points pair** (directly below the pupil) gently touch lower part of closed eyelids with your thumbs pointing inwards, ROLL the Client's eyelids (by rolling thumbs inwards) and HOLD it. (includes the **Madhya Vartma points pair** also (**Shringataka eyes extended**).

---

4 Nose+Lips Stages
42. Touch **i.) Phana marma points pair** touch lightly with both index fingers at 45° angle on either side of nose.
43. Touch **ii.) KapolaNasa marma points pair (Shringataka)** touch lightly with both index fingers at 90° angle on either side of nose.

44. Touch **iii.) Oshtha marma point (Shringataka tongue)** touch with your right index finger and roll the Client's skin there clockwise at an easy pace.
45. Touch **iv.) Hanu marma point (Shringataka tongue)** touch with your right index finger and roll the Client's skin there clockwise at an easy pace.

---

4 Cheek+Ear Stages
46. Touch **i.) Shankha marma points pair** (temples) touch lightly with both index fingers.
47. Touch **ii.) KapolaMadhya marma points pair (Shringataka tongue extended)** (at the depression in the cheek when we clench our teeth) touch lightly with both index fingers.
48. Touch **iii.) Karnapala marma points pair (Shringataka ears extended)** (top of earlobes) pinch and PULL firmly with thumb and index finger.
49. Touch **iv.) Karnapali marma points pair (Shringataka ears)** (bottom of earlobes where girls wear earrings) pinch and PUSH firmly with thumb and index finger.

---

3 Neck + 3 Throat Stages
50. Touch **i-a.) Manya (Mantha) marma points pair** (1/3rds of distance from top on sternocleidomastoid muscle that helps the neck to turn) touch lightly with both index fingers.
51. Touch **ii-a.) Nila (Sira Mantha) marma points pair** (2/3rds of distance from top on sternocleidomastoid muscle that helps the neck to turn) touch lightly with both index fingers.
52. Touch **iii-a.) Akshaka (Matrika) marma points pair** (base of sternocleidomastoid muscle that helps the neck to turn) touch lightly with both index fingers.
Note: This is very close to the Kanthanadi marma point which is in the center.

53. Touch **i-b.) Kantha (Matrika) marma point** (junction of head and neck) touch with your right index finger and roll the Client's skin there clockwise at an easy pace.
54. Touch **ii-b.) Sira Matrika marma point** (base of neck where it meets throat, base of adam's apple) touch with your right index finger and roll the Client's skin there clockwise at an easy pace.
55. Touch **iii-b.) Kanthanadi (Matrika) marma point** (depression below adam's apple) touch with your right index finger and roll the Client's skin there clockwise at an easy pace.
Note: This is very close to the Akshaka marma points on either side of it.

---

56. Now gently move to the right side of Client and take few deep breaths. Reestablish your silent Japa. Position yourself appropriately so your stance and breath are stable without strain.

4 Chest+Abdomen Midline Stages
57. Touch **i.) Jatru marma point (Hridaya extended**) (Manubrium breast bone at top of sternum) tap lightly 7 times with curved index finger. (*tap as in a knock on the door*).
58. Touch **ii.) Hridaya marma point** (depression below the sternum, esophageal orifice, inline with nipples) touch lightly with your right index finger and roll Client's skin clockwise at an easy pace.
59. Touch **iii.) Surya marma point (Hridaya extended**) (stomach two angula above nabhi) PRESS firmly with your right index finger and roll the Client's skin there clockwise at an easy pace.
60. Touch **iv.) Basti marma point** (bladder area two angula below nabhi) PRESS firmly with your right index finger and roll the Client's skin there clockwise at an easy pace.

Here ends the touch routine. Breathe calmly for few moments.

---

61. Glance at the clock and you may stretch yourself and have a sip of water and take a stroll for 10 minutes within visible/hearing range of Client.

62. Then sit again at the right side of the Client. Softly give them the instruction to roll over to the right side, then wait a few moments. Now give the instruction that they may slowly rise to a sitting position, and smilingly open the eyes at their own pace.

63. Parting pleasantries and instructions to have more water, juices and soups for the next couple of days. And to avoid social media.

Which? Suggested Oils Meditation

The Art of Living Sudarshan Kriya https://www.artofliving.org/in-en/sudarshan-kriya

Meditations by Sri Sri Ravi Shankar https://www.youtube.com/@MeditationsByGurudev

Ujjayi Pranayama https://www.artofliving.org/in-en/yoga/breathing-techniques/ujjayi-breathing

Brahmi Amla Oil https://www.sanjeevika.com/brahmi-amla-oil-200ml/

Ashwagandha Oil https://tae.in/products/varaasa-ashwanyam-ashwagandha-rich-body-oil
https://www.amazon.in/Zidella-Shilajit-Ashwagandha-Ayurvedic-Massage/dp/B0BHSGPBP4/

Mahanarayana Oil
https://www.amazon.in/Kerala-Ayurveda-Mahanarayana-Thailam-200/dp/B07F5M6217/

Almond Oil https://www.amazon.in/Hamdard-Roghan-Badam-Shirin-Almond/dp/B002MBG5MM/

Kshirabala Oil https://www.srisritattva.com/products/shop-kshirabala-taila-100ml

Dhanwantharam Oil https://www.keralaayurveda.biz/product/dhanwantharam-thailam

Anu Taila https://www.srisritattva.com/products/shop-anu-taila-10ml

Rose Scent Oil https://www.forestessentialsindia.com/after-bath-oil-indian-rose-absolute-new.html

Mustard Oil (highly pungent aroma)
https://www.amazon.in/Fortune-Kachi-Ghani-Pure-Mustard/dp/B0757631XR

Balm https://www.amazon.in/Zandu-Balm-25-ml/dp/B00J046NAI

Goghrit Sushma A+ (Noseghee) https://gosushma.wordpress.com/products/

Shakti Drops
https://www.srisritattva.com/collections/all-products/products/shop-shakti-drops-immunity-booster

Notes from personal Marma sessions

Year 2000 as Client
~March – During the annual Advanced Meditation courses at Rishikesh, an Englishman gave some of us Marma chikitsa, and I too benefitted.

Year 2004 as Client
~September – During the early days of our Ayurveda and Panchakarma setup, I frequented Mani Bhaiya's house in Bangalore Ashram (Ashwini-II kutir). Once I was lucky to get a marma touch from him, to heal my low back pain.

Year 2008 as Client
~July – When we were in Gujarat Ashram, Prasoon revealed that he was a Marma practitioner, and I received a session for tiredness and lack of sleep. At that time Vijaybhai also benefitted from a sore back.

Year 2017 as Client
~December – Jyoti had just learnt the exciting new siddha marma, and I was fortunate to get some touch therapy from her for headache and fever in Soudhamini flat.

Year 2020 as Client
November – I had severe Vata imbalance (caused by drinking cold fluids) leading to pain in almost every joint, especially in fingers. After three marma therapy sessions over three days, the pain became bearable and I could resume normal duties.

Year 2021 as Client
May – My vata imbalance had considerably reduced, however the joint stiffness persisted. After three marma sessions, the root cause got fully resolved, and after a couple of months, I recovered completely. I had also modified my diet, taking warm vegetable soups and soaked nuts, also chyawanprash and vitamins. Besides being regular in Sudarshan Kriya and Sahaj Samadhi meditation.

Year 2022 as Client
February – I took a marma session for aching neck and right shoulder. The neck pain got relieved, while the shoulder ache was reduced.

Year 2022 as Practitioner

- 22nd Sep Willey 7:30-8:30pm (*relief from guilt and fears*)
- 29th Sep Mahavir Mumma 3:45-4:30pm (*reported her severe right shoulder pain has considerably lessened*)
- 29th Sep Jaswinder 5:00-5:35pm *(dozed off easily*)
- 04th Oct Preeti 7:40-8:30am (*saw inner lights for the first time in a deep samadhi-like state*)
- 04th Oct Banka 9:00-10:00am (*peace and calmness*)
- 04th Oct Anuj 11:00-12noon (*strong tingling sensation at Medulla Oblongata manya mula point*)
- 04th Oct Anusha 8:30-9:30pm (*felt an hour passed in just a few minutes, so soon*)
- 06th Oct Jagjit 8:00-9:00pm (*during after dinner walk, felt a unique intimacy with nature, with plants and trees and stars*)

Etymology of word AYURVEDA

Sanskrit Grammar
Āyurveda = Āyur-Veda = sandhi of words, Āyus + Veda.

आयुर्वेदः = आयुर् वेदः = आयुः + वेदः ।

आयुः = Nominative Singular from neuter stem आयुस् ।

वेदः = Nominative Singular from masculine stem वेद ।

आयुः + वेदः = आयुर् वेदः by Sandhi in Grammar = आयुर्वेदः ।

आयुर्वेदः = Nominative Singular from masculine stem आयुर्वेद ।

In English we simply write the stem आयुर्वेद as Ayurveda.

Meaning

आयुस् = life, longevity, health, vivacity.

वेद = knowledge, system of knowing, precise information.

Thus, Ayurveda translates as the precise knowledge of life and well-being, a system of maintaining good health, curing and preventing illness, and enabling longevity of lifespan.

Āyurveda = the science of life, living well, wellness program

Latin Transliteration Chart

International Alphabet of Sanskrit Transliteration (I.A.S.T.)

a	ā	i	ī	u	ū	ṛ	ṝ	ḷ	
अ	आ	इ	ई	उ	ऊ	ऋ	ॠ	ऌ	
						◌ृ	◌ॄ	◌ॢ	
e	ai	o	au	ṃ	m̐	ḥ	Ardha Visarga	oṃ	
ए	ऐ	ओ	औ	◌ं	◌ँ	◌ः	ᳲ	ॐ	
Consonants shown with vowel 'a= अ' for uttering									
ka	क	ca	च	ṭa	ट	ta	त	pa	प
kha	ख	cha	छ	ṭha	ठ	tha	थ	pha	फ
ga	ग	ja	ज	ḍa	ड	da	द	ba	ब
gha	घ	jha	झ	ḍha	ढ	dha	ध	bha	भ
ṅa	ङ	ña	ञ	ṇa	ण	na	न	ma	म
ya	ra	la	va		ḷa	ʻ			
य	र	ल	व		ळ	ऽ			
							Consonant only		
śa	ṣa	sa	ha				ka	क्अ = क	
श	ष	स	ह				k	क्	

Marma Points List

Marma Point No	Sanskrit Name	English Name	
1,2	क्षिप्र	kṣipra (kshipra)	leg
3,4	तलहृदय	talahṛdaya (talahridaya)	leg
5,6	कूर्च	kūrca (kurcha)	leg
7,8	कूर्चशिर	kūrcaśira (kurchashira)	leg
9,10	गुल्फ	gulpha	leg
11,12	इन्द्रबस्ति	indrabasti	leg
13,14	जानु	jānu (janu)	leg
15,16	आणि	āṇi (ani)	leg
17,18	ऊर्वी	ūrvī (urvi)	leg
19,20	लोहिताक्ष	lohitākṣa (lohitaksha)	leg
21,22	विटप	viṭapa (vitapa)	leg
23,24	क्षिप्र	kṣipra (kshipra)	arm
25,26	तलहृदय	talahṛdaya (talahridaya)	arm
27,28	कूर्च	kūrca (kurcha)	arm
29,30	कूर्चशिर	kūrcaśira (kurchashira)	arm
31,32	मणिबन्ध	maṇibandha (manibandha)	arm
33,34	इन्द्रबस्ति	indrabasti	arm
35,36	कूर्पर	kūrpara (kurpara)	arm
37,38	आणि	āṇi (ani)	arm
39,40	ऊर्वी / बाह्वी	ūrvī (urvi) / bāhvī	arm
41,42	लोहिताक्ष	lohitākṣa (lohitaksha)	arm
43,44	कक्षधर	kakṣadhara (kakshadhara)	arm
45	गुद	guda	
46	बस्ति	basti	
47	नाभि	nābhi (nabhi)	
48	हृदय	hṛdaya (hridaya)	
49,50	स्तनमूल	stanamūla (stanamula)	
51,52	स्तनरोहित	stanarohita	
53,54	अपलाप	apalāpa (apalapa)	
55,56	अपस्तम्भ	apastambha	
57,58	कटीकतरुण	kaṭīkataruṇa (katikataruna)	
59,60	कुकुन्दर	kukundara	

61,62	नितम्ब	nitamba
63,64	पार्श्वसन्धि	pārśvasandhi (parshvasandhi)
65,66	बृहती	bṛhatī (brihati)
67,68	अंसफलक	aṃsaphalaka (amsaphalaka)
69,70	अंस	aṃsa (amsa)
71,72	धमनी नीला / सिरामन्थ	dhamanī nīlā (nila) / sirāmantha
73,74	धमनी मन्या / मन्थ	dhamanī / manyā (manya) mantha
75,76	मातृका अक्षक 1a, 1b	mātṛkā akshaka 1a, 1b (matrika akshaka)
77	मातृका कण्ठनाडी 2a	mātṛkā kaṇṭhanāḍī 2a (matrika kanthanadi)
78	मातृका कण्ठ 2b	mātṛkā kaṇṭha 2b (matrika kantha)
79,80	मातृका पृष्ठग्रीव 3a, 3b	mātṛkā pṛṣṭhagrīva 3a, 3b (matrika prishtagriva)
81	मातृका मन्यामणि 4a	mātṛkā manyāmaṇi 4a (matrika manyamani)
82	मातृका ग्रीवा 4b	mātṛkā grīvā 4b (matrika griva)
83,84	कृकाटिका	kṛkāṭikā (krikatika)
85,86	विधुर	vidhura
87,88	फण	phaṇa (phana)
89,90	अपाङ्ग	apāṅga (apanga)
91,92	आवर्त	āvarta (avarta)
93,94	शङ्ख	śaṅkha (shankha)
95,96	उत्क्षेप	utkṣepa (utkshepa)
97	स्थपनी	sthapanī (sthapani)
98	शृङ्गाटक जिह्वा 1a = ओष्ठ, 1b = हनु	śṛṅgāṭaka 1 oṣṭha, hanu (shringataka oshtha, hanu)
99	शृङ्गाटक घ्राण 2a,b = कपोल नासा	śṛṅgāṭaka 2 kapolanāsā (shringataka kapolanasa)
100	शृङ्गाटक श्रोत्र 3a,b = कर्णपालि	śṛṅgāṭaka 3 karṇapāli (shringataka karnapali)
101	शृङ्गाटक अक्षि 4a,b = कनीनका	śṛṅgāṭaka 4 kanīnakā (shringataka kaninaka)
102	सीमन्त 1 = नासामूल	sīmanta 1 nāsāmūla (simanta nasamula)
103	सीमन्त 2 = कपाल	sīmanta 2 kapāla (simanta kapala)
104	सीमन्त 3 = विष्णुरन्ध्र	sīmanta 3 viṣṇurandhra (simanta vishnurandhra)
105	सीमन्त 4 = शिवरन्ध्र	sīmanta 4 śivarandhra (simanta shivarandhra)
106	सीमन्त 5 = मन्यामूल	sīmanta 5 manyāmūla (simanta manyamula)
107	अधिपति (ब्रह्मरंध्र / मूर्ध्नि)	adhipati (brahmarandhra or mūrdhni or crown)

Note: The Marma Point No is an arbitrary number used herein for clarity.

Index of Marma Points Sanskrit

Sanskrit Name		English Name		Marma Point No
अंस		aṃsa (amsa)		69,70
अंसफलक		aṃsaphalaka (amsaphalaka)		67,68
अधिपति (ब्रह्मरंध्र / मूर्ध्नि)		adhipati (brahmarandhra or mūrdhni or crown)		107
अपलाप		apalāpa (apalapa)		53,54
अपस्तम्भ		apastambha		55,56
अपाङ्ग		apāṅga (apanga)		89,90
आणि	पाद	āṇi (ani)	leg	15,16
आणि	बाहु	āṇi (ani)	arm	37,38
आवर्त		āvarta (avarta)		91,92
इन्द्रबस्ति	पाद	indrabasti	leg	11,12
इन्द्रबस्ति	बाहु	indrabasti	arm	33,34
उत्क्षेप		utkṣepa (utkshepa)		95,96
ऊर्वी	पाद	ūrvī (urvi)	leg	17,18
ऊर्वी / बाह्वी	बाहु	ūrvī (urvi) / bāhvī	arm	39,40
कक्षधर		kakṣadhara (kakshadhara)		43,44
कटीकतरुण		kaṭīkataruṇa (katikataruna)		57,58
कुकुन्दर		kukundara		59,60
कूर्च	पाद	kūrca (kurcha)	leg	5,6
कूर्च	बाहु	kūrca (kurcha)	arm	27,28
कूर्चशिर	पाद	kūrcaśira (kurchashira)	leg	7,8
कूर्चशिर	बाहु	kūrcaśira (kurchashira)	arm	29,30
कूर्पर		kūrpara (kurpara)		35,36
कृकाटिका		kṛkāṭikā (krikatika)		83,84
क्षिप्र	पाद	kṣipra (kshipra)	leg	1,2
क्षिप्र	बाहु	kṣipra (kshipra)	arm	23,24
गुद		guda		45
गुल्फ		gulpha		9,10
जानु		jānu (janu)		13,14
तलहृदय	पाद	talahṛdaya (talahridaya)	leg	3,4
तलहृदय	बाहु	talahṛdaya (talahridaya)	arm	25,26
धमनी मन्या / मन्थ		dhamanī manyā (manya) / mantha		73,74
धमनी नीला / सिरामन्थ		dhamanī nīlā (nila) / sirāmantha		71,72

नाभि		nābhi (nabhi)		47
नितम्ब		nitamba		61,62
पार्श्वसन्धि		pārśvasandhi (parshvasandhi)		63,64
फण		phaṇa (phana)		87,88
बस्ति		basti		46
बृहती		bṛhatī (brihati)		65,66
मणिबन्ध		maṇibandha (manibandha)		31,32
मातृका अक्षक 1a, 1b		mātṛkā akshaka 1a, 1b (matrika akshaka)		75,76
मातृका कण्ठ 2b		mātṛkā kaṇṭha 2b (matrika kantha)		78
मातृका कण्ठनाडी 2a		mātṛkā kaṇṭhanāḍī 2a (matrika kanthanadi)		77
मातृका ग्रीवा 4b		mātṛkā grīvā 4b (matrika griva)		82
मातृका पृष्ठग्रीव 3a, 3b		mātṛkā pṛṣṭhagrīva 3a, 3b (matrika prishtagriva)		79,80
मातृका मन्यामणि 4a		mātṛkā manyāmaṇi 4a (matrika manyamani)		81
लोहिताक्ष	पाद	lohitākṣa (lohitaksha)	leg	19,20
लोहिताक्ष	बाहु	lohitākṣa (lohitaksha)	arm	41,42
विटप		viṭapa (vitapa)		21,22
विधुर		vidhura		85,86
शङ्ख		śaṅkha (shankha)		93,94
शृङ्गाटक अक्षि 4a,b = कनीनका		śṛṅgāṭaka 4 kanīnakā (shringataka kaninaka)		101
शृङ्गाटक घ्राण 2a,b = कपोल नासा		śṛṅgāṭaka 2 kapolanāsā (shringataka kapolanasa)		99
शृङ्गाटक जिह्वा 1a = ओष्ठ, 1b = हनु		śṛṅgāṭaka 1 oṣṭha, hanu (shringataka oshtha, hanu)		98
शृङ्गाटक श्रोत्र 3a,b = कर्णपालि		śṛṅgāṭaka 3 karṇapāli (shringataka karnapali)		100
सीमन्त 1 = नासामूल		sīmanta 1 nāsāmūla (simanta nasamula)		102
सीमन्त 2 = कपाल		sīmanta 2 kapāla (simanta kapala)		103
सीमन्त 3 = विष्णुरन्ध्र		sīmanta 3 viṣṇurandhra (simanta vishnurandhra)		104
सीमन्त 4 = शिवरन्ध्र		sīmanta 4 śivarandhra (simanta shivarandhra)		105
सीमन्त 5 = मन्यामूल		sīmanta 5 manyāmūla (simanta manyamula)		106
स्तनमूल		stanamūla (stanamula)		49,50
स्तनरोहित		stanarohita		51,52
स्थपनी		sthapanī (sthapani)		97
हृदय		hṛdaya (hridaya)		48

Note: The Marma Point No is an arbitrary number used herein for clarity.

Index of Marma Points English

English Name		Sanskrit Name	Marma Point No
adhipati (brahmarandhra or mūrdhni or crown)		अधिपति (ब्रह्मरंध्र / मूर्ध्नि)	107
aṃsa (amsa)		अंस	69,70
aṃsaphalaka (amsaphalaka)		अंसफलक	67,68
āṇi (ani)	leg	आणि	15,16
āṇi (ani)	arm	आणि	37,38
apalāpa (apalapa)		अपलाप	53,54
apāṅga (apanga)		अपाङ्ग	89,90
apastambha		अपस्तम्भ	55,56
āvarta (avarta)		आवर्त	91,92
basti		बस्ति	46
bṛhatī (brihati)		बृहती	65,66
dhamanī nīlā (nila) / sirāmantha		धमनी नीला / सिरामन्थ	71,72
dhamanī manyā (manya) / mantha		धमनी मन्या / मन्थ	73,74
guda		गुद	45
gulpha		गुल्फ	9,10
hṛdaya (hridaya)		हृदय	48
indrabasti	leg	इन्द्रबस्ति	11,12
indrabasti	arm	इन्द्रबस्ति	33,34
jānu (janu)		जानु	13,14
kakṣadhara (kakshadhara)		कक्षधर	43,44
kaṭīkataruṇa (katikataruna)		कटीकतरुण	57,58
kṛkāṭikā (krikatika)		कृकाटिका	83,84
kṣipra (kshipra)	leg	क्षिप्र	1,2
kṣipra (kshipra)	arm	क्षिप्र	23,24
kukundara		कुकुन्दर	59,60
kūrca (kurcha)	leg	कूर्च	5,6
kūrca (kurcha)	arm	कूर्च	27,28
kūrcaśira (kurchashira)	leg	कूर्चशिर	7,8
kūrcaśira (kurchashira)	arm	कूर्चशिर	29,30
kūrpara (kurpara)		कूर्पर	35,36

lohitākṣa (lohitaksha)	leg	लोहिताक्ष	19,20
lohitākṣa (lohitaksha)	arm	लोहिताक्ष	41,42
maṇibandha (manibandha)		मणिबन्ध	31,32
mātṛkā akshaka 1a, 1b (matrika akshaka)		मातृका अक्षक 1a, 1b	75,76
mātṛkā grīvā 4b (matrika griva)		मातृका ग्रीवा 4b	82
mātṛkā kaṇṭha 2b (matrika kantha)		मातृका कण्ठ 2b	78
mātṛkā kaṇṭhanāḍī 2a (matrika kanthanadi)		मातृका कण्ठनाडी 2a	77
mātṛkā manyāmaṇi 4a (matrika manyamani)		मातृका मन्यामणि 4a	81
mātṛkā pṛṣṭhagrīva 3a, 3b (matrika prishtagriva)		मातृका पृष्ठग्रीव 3a, 3b	79,80
nābhi (nabhi)		नाभि	47
nitamba		नितम्ब	61,62
pārśvasandhi (parshvasandhi)		पार्श्वसन्धि	63,64
phaṇa (phana)		फण	87,88
śaṅkha (shankha)		शङ्ख	93,94
sīmanta 1 nāsāmūla (simanta nasamula)		सीमन्त 1 = नासामूल	102
sīmanta 2 kapāla (simanta kapala)		सीमन्त 2 = कपाल	103
sīmanta 3 viṣṇurandhra (simanta vishnurandhra)		सीमन्त 3 = विष्णुरन्ध्र	104
sīmanta 4 śivarandhra (simanta shivarandhra)		सीमन्त 4 = शिवरन्ध्र	105
sīmanta 5 manyāmūla (simanta manyamula)		सीमन्त 5 = मन्यामूल	106
śṛṅgāṭaka 1 oṣṭha, hanu (shringataka oshtha, hanu)		शृङ्गाटक जिह्वा 1a = ओष्ठ, 1b = हनु	98
śṛṅgāṭaka 2 kapolanāsā (shringataka kapolanasa)		शृङ्गाटक घ्राण 2a,b = कपोल नासा	99
śṛṅgāṭaka 3 karṇapāli (shringataka karnapali)		शृङ्गाटक श्रोत्र 3a,b = कर्णपालि	100
śṛṅgāṭaka 4 kanīnakā (shringataka kaninaka)		शृङ्गाटक अक्षि 4a,b = कनीनका	101
stanamūla (stanamula)		स्तनमूल	49,50
stanarohita		स्तनरोहित	51,52
sthapanī (sthapani)		स्थपनी	97
talahṛdaya (talahridaya)	leg	तलहृदय	3,4
talahṛdaya (talahridaya)	arm	तलहृदय	25,26
ūrvī (urvi)	leg	ऊर्वी	17,18
ūrvī (urvi) / bāhvī	arm	ऊर्वी / बाह्वी	39,40
utkṣepa (utkshepa)		उत्क्षेप	95,96
vidhura		विधुर	85,86
viṭapa (vitapa)		विटप	21,22

Note: The Marma Point No is an arbitrary number used herein for clarity.

Few Marma Points named variously

Here is a table of marma points that have been named differently by various authors.

English Name		Sanskrit Name		Marma Point No
adhipati (brahmarandhra / mūrdhni) (called vishnurandhra by some)		अधिपति (ब्रह्मरंध्र / मूर्ध्नि)		107
nīlā / sirāmantha		नीला / सिरामन्थ		71,72
manyā / mantha		मन्या / मन्थ		73,74
mātṛkā / sirāmātṛkā		मातृका / सिरामातृका		75,76
ūrvī (urvi) / bāhvī	arm	ऊर्वी / बाह्वी	बाहु	39,40

Marma points that are not explicitly named in Samhita, but by some authors for clarity

English Name	Sanskrit Name	Marma Point No
mātṛkā 1a, 1b (akshaka)	मातृका अक्षक 1a, 1b	75,76
mātṛkā 2a (kaṇṭhanāḍī)	मातृका कण्ठनाडी 2a	77
mātṛkā 2b (kaṇṭha)	मातृका कण्ठ 2b	78
mātṛkā 3a, 3b (pṛṣṭhagrīva)	मातृका पृष्ठग्रीव 3a, 3b	79,80
mātṛkā 4a (manyāmaṇi)	मातृका मन्यामणि 4a	81
mātṛkā 4b (grīvā)	मातृका ग्रीवा 4b	82
śṛṅgāṭaka 1 (oṣṭha, hanu)	श्रृङ्गाटक जिह्वा 1a = ओष्ठ, 1b = हनु	98
śṛṅgāṭaka 2 (kapolanāsā)	श्रृङ्गाटक घ्राण 2a,b = कपोलनासा	99
śṛṅgāṭaka 3 (karṇapāli)	श्रृङ्गाटक श्रोत्र 3a,b = कर्णपालि	100
śṛṅgāṭaka 4 (kanīnakā)	श्रृङ्गाटक अक्षि 4a,b = कनीनका	101
sīmanta 1 (nāsāmūla)	सीमन्त 1 = नासामूल	102
sīmanta 2 (kapāla)	सीमन्त 2 = कपाल	103
sīmanta 3 (viṣṇurandhra)	सीमन्त 3 = विष्णुरन्ध्र	104
sīmanta 4 (śivarandhra)	सीमन्त 4 = शिवरन्ध्र	105
sīmanta 5 (manyāmūla)	सीमन्त 5 = मन्यामूल	106

References

https://www.ashtangayoga.info/philosophy/sanskrit-and-devanagari/transliteration-tool/#devanagari/iast/
https://www.learnsanskrit.cc/

https://niimh.nic.in/ebooks/ecaraka/?mod=adhi
https://www.nhp.gov.in/marma-therapy_mtl
https://www.srisritattvapanchakarma.com/meru-chikitsa/
https://www.srisritattvapanchakarma.com/product/marma/
https://sscasrh.org/panchakarma/
https://artoflivingretreatcenter.org/blog/revathi-raghavan-marma/
https://www.facebook.com/ArtofLivingUSA/posts/marma-therapy-an-important-part-of-ayurveda-that-helps-to-maintain-health-by-cle/10157648714167437/
https://artoflivingretreatcenter.org/blog/revathi-raghavan-marma/

Marmas of the Head and Neck
https://www.easyayurveda.com/2017/06/15/head-neck-marma/

Seat of Prana
https://vaidyanamah.com/marma/

Charaka Siddhisthana Chapter 9 Tri Marmiya Siddhi
https://www.easyayurveda.com/2023/03/17/charaka-siddhisthana-9-tri-marmiya/

Facial Marma Therapy with Nefertiti
https://www.youtube.com/watch?v=Isbux8cApQ4

Marma Chikitsa Points for Balanced Emotions
https://www.youtube.com/watch?v=BMjmoIZY784

Ayurvedic Indian Marma Points for Head Massage
https://www.youtube.com/watch?v=VBk-3W0e0v4

Rudram Chants for gentle Marma stimulation
https://www.youtube.com/watch?v=PbGBn14Q-TU

Guided Meditations Sri Sri Ravi Shankar
Chakras & Our Unseen Bodies
https://www.youtube.com/watch?v=0iZA70Eri98

Day 1 of the 21 Day Meditation
https://www.youtube.com/watch?v=v1vRphAv7C4

Vasant Lad – Marma Points of Ayurveda – 1st – 2015 – Ayurvedic Press, New Mexico.

Vasant Lad – Applied Marma Therapy Cards – 2nd – 2014 – Ayurvedic Press, New Mexico.

Ernst Schrott – Marma Therapy : The Healing Power of Ayurvedic Vital Point Massage – 1st – 2016 – Singing Dragon, London.

Frawley Ranade Lele – Ayurveda and Marma Therapy – 1st – 2003 – Lotus Press, Wisconsin.

Swami Omkarmurti Saraswati – Marma Yoga Vol1 – 1st – 2020 – Yoga Publications Trust, Munger.

Binod Kumar Joshi – Ayurvedic Healing Methods Marma Chikitsa – 1st – 2021 – Motilal Banarsidass Publications, Delhi.

John Chitty – Energy Exercises: Easy Exercises for Health and Vitality – 2nd – 2018 – CSES Colorado School of Energy Studies, Boulder.

Richard Gordon – Quantum Touch – 1st – 2006 – North Atlantic Books, Berkeley California.

Franklyn Sills – The Polarity Process – 1st – 2001 – North Atlantic Books, Berkeley California.

John Beaulieu – Polarity Therapy Workbook – 2nd – 2016 – Biosonics, New York.

Amadea Morningstar – The Ayurvedic Guide to Polarity Therapy – 1st – 2001 – Lotus Press, Wisconsin.

Acharya Balkrishna – अष्टाङ्गहृदयम् (सूत्र स्थानम्) – 1st – 2014 – Divya Prakashan, Patanjali Yogpeeth Haridwar.

Anant Ram Sharma – सुश्रुत संहिता (शारीर स्थानम्) – 1st – 2021 – Chaukhamba Surbharati Prakashan, Varanasi.

Atrideva – सुश्रुत संहिता (संपूर्ण संस्कृत-हिंदी टीका) – 1st – 2015 – Motilal Banarsidass Publishing House, New Delhi.

K R Srikantha Murthy – Illustrated Sushruta Samhita Vol1 – 1st Reprint – 2022 – Chaukhamba Orientalia, Varanasi.

Sanjay Pisharodi – Acharya Vagbhata's Astanga Hridayam Vol1 Chapters 1 to 4 – 1st 2016 – Purnarogya Holistic Healing Centre, Kerala.

T Sreekumar – Astanga Hridaya Vagbhata Sutrasthana Vol 1 & 2 – 7th - 2018 – Harisree Publications, Kerala.

P V Sharma – Caraka Samhita Vol II Chikitsasthana Kalpasthana Siddhisthana – 4th - 1998 – Chaukhambha Orientalia, Varanasi.

Epilogue

White or Non-White, Man's inner color is both and neither. White light splits into seven colors of a rainbow to indicate the seven continents and seven oceans, i.e., all of humanity. Black or Dark hair is as attractive as red or blonde.

Take your pick, someday you shall know Two as One.

सर्वे भवन्तु सुखिनः । सर्वे सन्तु निरामयाः ।

सर्वे भद्राणि पश्यन्तु । मा कश्चिद् दुःख भाग्भवेत् ॥

ॐ शान्तिः शान्तिः शान्तिः ॥

When faith has blossomed in life,
Every step is led by the Divine.

Sri Sri Ravi Shankar

Om Namah Shivaya

जय गुरुदेव

www.ingramcontent.com/pod-product-compliance
Lightning Source LLC
LaVergne TN
LVHW070437070526
838199LV00015B/533
* 9 7 8 9 3 9 5 7 6 6 0 7 4 *